Face to face with distress:
the professional use of self in

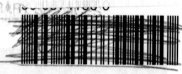

Face to face with distress:
the professional use of self in psychosocial care

Edited by

Peter Griffiths, BSc(Hons)Soc/Psy SRN RMN
Clinical Nurse Specialist, Research and Development,
the Cassel Hospital, Richmond, Surrey, UK

Jacqueline Ord, SRN BA PhD
Research Fellow, Directorate of Public Health and Clinical Policy,
North Essex Health Authority, UK

Diane Wells, SRN BA DipSocStud DN (London) DipSocRes CertEd RNT
Lecturer, Faculty of Health Care Sciences, Kingston University and
St George's Hospital Medical School, London, UK

Consultant Editor

Elizabeth Barnes, SRN
Former nurse at the Cassel Hospital, Richmond, Surrey, UK

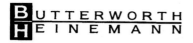

Butterworth-Heinemann
Linacre House, Jordan Hill, Oxford OX2 8DP
A division of Reed International and Professional Publishing Ltd

℟ A member of the Reed Elsevier plc group

OXFORD   BOSTON   JOHANNESBURG
MELBOURNE   NEW DELHI   SINGAPORE

First published 1998

British Library Cataloguing in Publication Data
A catalogue record for this book is available from the British Library

Library of Congress Cataloguing in Publication Data
A catalogue record for this book is available from the Library of Congress

ISBN 0 7506 3617 3

Typeset by AFS Image Setters Ltd, Glasgow
and printed and bound in Great Britain by Biddles Ltd, Guildford and Kings Lynn

Contents

Contributors   ix

Foreword   xiii
Christine Hancock

Preface   xv
Elizabeth Barnes

Acknowledgements   xix

Section One: Models and frameworks   1

Introduction   3
Peter Griffiths

Chapter 1
Psychosocial nursing: a model learnt from experience   5
Peter Griffiths and George Leach
    Part 1
    The Cassel Hospital: history and current practice   5
    Part 2
    Making explicit the Cassel model   11

Chapter 2
Subjective experience and social enquiry   42
Jacqueline Ord

Chapter 3
Implementing change: lessons learnt from the Cassel Hospital/
Austen Riggs Center exchange programme   53
Mimi Francis

Chapter 4
National policy and professional practice   59
Gillian Chapman

Section Two: Practice   67

Introduction   69
Jacqueline Ord

Chapter 5
The use of leisure activities in psychosocial nursing   71
Graham McCaffrey

Chapter 6
Nursing an adult survivor of childhood sexual abuse   83
Fritha Irwin

Chapter 7
The use of self in child protection work   95
Vicki Mills

Chapter 8
Mary's story   108
Ann Simpson

Chapter 9
Pain as memory   119
Gillian Parker

Chapter 10
Knowing patients: how much and how well?   135
Louise de Raeve

Section Three: Developing the practitioner   147

Introduction   149
Diane Wells

Chapter 11
Psychosexual nursing seminars   152
Doreen Clifford

Chapter 12
How can I help?   163
Charlie McGrory

Chapter 13
Biographical work with older people   178
Diane Wells

Chapter 14
Clinical supervision   188
Mic Rafferty

Chapter 15
Psychosocial issues of racism in the caring professions:
a black perspective   198
Sonia Stephen

Chapter 16
Learning through experience   210
Louise de Lambert

Index   223

Contributors

Elizabeth Barnes (Lucas), SRN, nursed at the Cassel Hospital from 1951 to 1957. She won the *Nursing Times* Golden Jubilee Journalism Bursary and worked for the journal for two years. She co-ordinated an international study on human relations in general hospitals for the World Federation for Mental Health (*People in Hospital*, Macmillan, 1961). She was appointed Matron of the Henderson Hospital (1961–1966) and acted as psychosocial nursing consultant at the Ulleväl Sykehus, Oslo. She worked for the Kings's Fund as a team member of the Hospitals Internal Communications Project, as a tutor at the Ward Sisters' College, and for 10 years, until retirement, as Publications and Press Secretary. Elizabeth Barnes was the editor of the first book about psychosocial nursing from the Cassel Hospital (*Psychosocial Nursing*, Tavistock, 1968).

Gillian Chapman, RGN, RSCN, BSc, MSc, PhD, is Assistant Chief Nursing Officer, heading up the Nursing Strategy and Policy Development Unit in the Department of Health. She has been with the Department since 1989, and her responsibilities have included children's services, public health, *Caring for people*, and working on *A vision for the future* and *The challenges for nursing and midwifery in the 21st century*. She was previously a lecturer in nursing at King's College, London, a director of nursing services for mental health, and worked at the Cassel Hospital from 1972 to 1976.

Doreen Clifford, SRN, SCM, MTD, was Matron of the Cassel Hospital from 1966 to 1975. Since 1963, she has been running seminars for a variety of care-workers including general nurses, residential social workers, nurse teachers, clergy and nurse counsellors. Since 1972, she has focused on seminars in psychosexual nursing for practitioners in all nursing specialties.

Mimi Francis, RN, MA, is an American nurse who received her master's degree in nursing from the University of Hawaii before undertaking the Cassel Hospital course. She worked at the Austen Riggs Center in Stockbridge, Massachusetts, for 10 years. She is currently working in Vermont as a psychiatric nurse practitioner with a range of clients including elderly people, prisoners and individuals in the community. She also provides consultation to nursing staff in various health care institutions.

Peter Griffiths, BSc, SRN, RMN, has had a career within the UK National Health Service spanning 20 years of clinical and managerial practice. He is currently Clinical Nurse Specialist for Research and Development at the Cassel Hospital, and has a particular interest in developing psychosocial practice in other health care settings through consultancy, courses and training. He is a visiting lecturer at the Tavistock Clinic and a member of the editorial board of the journal *Therapeutic Communities*.

Fritha Irwin, SRN, SCM, is a clinical nurse specialist for the therapeutic community team at the Cassel Hospital, where she has worked for seven years.

Louise de Lambert, RN, BAP, is from New Zealand, where she qualified as a psychiatric nurse, and then worked at Ashburn Hall, Dunedin. She joined the Cassel Hospital in 1968, and became Matron there in 1974. She completed psychotherapy training with the British Association of Psychotherapists in 1982, and now works in Auckland, New Zealand, as a psychotherapist, supervisor and consultant to professionals in mental health services.

George Leach, MA(Psychol), RMN, RGN, RNT, PGCE, Diploma in Advanced Psychodynamic Counselling, worked at the Cassel Hospital for five years, and for four years as an adviser on HIV to the World Health Organization. He returned to the Cassel as a part-time nurse tutor in 1993 to co-ordinate the redevelopment and accreditation of the Diploma in Psychosocial Nursing. He is currently working in private practice.

Graham McCaffrey, RGN, BSc, worked at the Cassel Hospital for six years. He worked on the community team, and was senior nurse on both single adult and families units. He is now living in Calgary, Canada.

Charlie McGrory, RMN, DN, BSc, worked at the Cassel Hospital from 1980 to 1992. He is Senior Lecturer, Mental Health Nursing, Wolfson School of Health Sciences, Thames Valley University.

Vicki Mills, SRN, CQSW, is currently a senior social worker, specializing in child protection.

Jacqueline Ord, SRN, BA, PhD, is Research Fellow at the Directorate of Public Health and Clinical Policy of North Essex Health Authority, and practises independently as a consultant in organizational development. She has worked at the Tavistock Institute of Human Relations as a researcher/consultant, and as a lecturer in management at Richmond College in London. She nursed at the Cassel Hospital from 1972 to 1977.

Gillian Parker, SRN, SCM psychoanalyst, Founder and Director of the Inner-City Centre, and Dean of Studies at the Lincoln Centre and Institute of Psychotherapy. She has worked on research and training projects at both the Cassel and Henderson hospitals, and has pioneered work in family therapy. She has worked on the advanced programme at the Tavistock Clinic and acted as supervisor to victim support schemes and to Cruse. She trained originally as a nurse, and worked with the Red Cross in Ethiopia during the Second World War. She now works for POPAN (Prevention of Professional Abuse Network).

Louise de Raeve, BA, RGN, Postgraduate Diploma in the Ethics of Health Care, is a general nurse who has worked at the Cassel Hospital and in the voluntary sector for an independent living scheme for physically disabled people. She has been teaching since 1989, including five years as McMillan Lecturer in Nursing Ethics at the University of Wales in Swansea, where she is currently a lecturer in the Department of Nursing, Midwifery and Health Care.

Mic Rafferty, RMN, worked at the Cassel Hospital from 1972 to 1980. He is currently programme manager for clinical development at the Department of Nursing, Midwifery and Health Care at the University of Wales, Swansea.

Ann Simpson, RGN, has worked in London, Switzerland and the USA, specializing in intensive care nursing. She has worked in mental health since 1977, both in the NHS and in the voluntary sector. Her current post is Senior Nurse Specialist and Nurse Adviser for the North Essex Child and Family Consultation Service.

Sonia Stephen, RHN, RMN, Dip Group Psych (London), MA Black Therapy (Hon)(née Francis) is a psychotherapist and black mental health specialist. She is co-director of the Black Therapy Diploma Course, and works for Lambeth Health Care Trust and in private practice.

Diane Wells (née Macklin), SRN, BA, Dip Soc Stud, DN (London), Dip Soc Res, Cert Ed, RNT, is a lecturer specializing in psychodynamic approaches for developing nursing care. After working as a sister and tutor at the Cassel Hospital from 1973 to 1981, she returned to teaching general nurses. She has held posts at the Royal Free Hospital School of Nursing, St Bartholomew's College of Nursing, and is now in the Faculty of Health Care Sciences, Kingston University and St George's Hospital Medical School. Her current research is concerned with developing nursing through biographical work with older people.

Foreword

Christine Hancock General Secretary, Royal College of Nursing

The psychosocial approach outlined in this book demonstrates nursing at its best, and offers all careworkers a creative and thoughtful way of dealing with the personal impact of their work. Nurses in many settings deal with people at their most vulnerable; they are literally face-to-face with distress on a daily basis, and their insight into the lives of the people they care for is an intimate one. Mental health nursing in particular, faces head-on some of the most difficult and uncomfortable issues we have to address as a society.

Nursing, paradoxically, has inherited a culture which in the past discouraged much thinking about feelings and emotions. Nurses and other health professionals may feel uneasy about using psychodynamic approaches in their work, and the relationship between psychodynamic theory and nursing is not clearly defined. Yet such approaches can provide a basis for understanding and working with difficult emotions, both in their patients and in themselves. From a psychodynamic perspective, this traditional resistance to thinking and feeling rather than doing can be seen as an understandable defence against continuous exposure to painful situations.

There are, however, a growing number of nurses who are pioneering new approaches; for example, liaison groups of mental health nurses who are providing consultancy to general nursing colleagues on dealing with distressed patients, and also those nurses developing choice in services for people with mental illness.

The model of care and learning which has evolved over the last five decades at the Cassel Hospital demonstrates the key role of nurses in meeting the needs of people who are confronting distress. The approach is both holistic and rigorous. It offers a way of 'doing' which is enriched by theoretical and emotional insight. Access to psychosocial nurse training needs to be more widely available; I hope this book will help that come about.

Preface

Psychosocial nursing began in the psychoanalytically-based therapeutic community at the Cassel Hospital soon after the Second World War. Since then, the hospital's staff have been influencing the thinking and practice of care-workers in hospitals, community health and other services, in teaching, research and the management of change. As a therapeutic community, the hospital attempts to turn experience into learning, using the everyday interaction of patients and staff as the focus of enquiry.

Our definition of 'care-worker' embraces all those who, during their everyday work, come face to face with people in distress. As well as nurses, it includes social workers, hospital doctors, general practitioners, counsellors, voluntary workers, paramedics and rescue workers, personnel managers, police officers, probation officers, prison officers, and clergy. And people in distress include not only individual psychiatric patients but also dysfunctional families; troubled youngsters at school, at home, and on the street; bereaved people; the victims and perpetrators of abuse and violence; people with grave medical disorders; and people distressed at work or by unemployment.

Everyone faces distress in the course of a lifetime. Some can deal with it in a private, personal way or with the help of family and friends. But many cannot. This book is intended to give care-workers who are involved with those many distressed people some help in thinking about new ways of developing their professional skills. It is not a 'how to' book. It is not a textbook. It describes the principles, practice and teaching of psychosocial nursing which nurses at the Cassel Hospital and outside have found useful. Not all the chapters describe success. It is perhaps from less successful ventures, even failures, that we can learn most.

A first comprehensive attempt to explain this new kind of nursing was a collection of chiefly reprinted papers by Tom Main, then Medical Director, Doreen Weddell, then Matron, and some of the nursing staff (Barnes 1968). This present volume, unlike the first, comprises hitherto unpublished work written entirely by the nurses.

It is divided into three sections: models and frameworks, practice, and development of the practitioner. The first section starts with the psycho-social model developed from practice and research at the hospital. It goes on to discuss the relevance of these ideas for organizational change and research, and for government health policy in the UK. The second section (practice) gives examples from the work of nurses in the hospital and in other care services; and the third (development of the practitioner) includes methods derived from the hospital's experience and used in other settings.

The divisions are artificial. The three sections comprise a triangle in which each 'angle' informs the other two and by which each learns from the other two. Unlike some other attempts at developing models, the Cassel model described here comes from practice which, in turn, becomes understandable through teaching and supervision.

Throughout this process, and from whichever angle we begin, is the underlying principle that the practitioner's own feelings that are aroused in work with distressed people can be used in a practical therapeutic way, both to understand the interaction and to hone the practitioner's skill. It is not only a matter of relieving the practitioner's distress, and that of the patient or client, important though that is. But, more important is to understand the distress and to learn how to use that understanding constructively. The emotional work of examining one's own feelings is usually painful. It requires courage, sensitivity, and an ability to articulate. Above all, it requires a safe, reliable support system maintained by the supervisor or teacher and the peer group. It also requires time to explore, and often to re-explore, the interaction and the feelings aroused, to enhance learning. These requirements need to be built into the organization's system of working, in other words, the framework within which people – care-workers and patients or clients – learn and work.

These matters are discussed in the following chapters by nurses who have been and are still going through that process. Readers who wish to follow up the ideas presented here are advised to write to the authors, either through the publisher, or care of the secretary of the Cassel Nurses' Association (The Cassel Hospital, 1 Ham Common, Richmond, Surrey TW10 7JF, UK).

Elizabeth Barnes

Reference

Barnes, E. ed. (1968). *Psychosocial Nursing: Studies from the Cassel Hospital.* Tavistock Publications.

Acknowledgements

We wish to thank the many people who have made this book possible: the authors who have struggled to put their ideas into print, and the people whose stories they tell; the Cassel Hospital, Richmond College, and North Essex Health Authority for their support and the use of their office facilities; and the Cassel Nurses' Association, of which this editorial team is a part, for their unfailing support. Special thanks to Susan Devlin, Butterworth-Heinemann, for her early interest and her continuing involvement, skill and patience.

Elizabeth Barnes
Peter Griffiths
Jacqueline Ord
Diane Wells

Section One

Models and frameworks

Introduction

Peter Griffiths

In this section on models and frameworks, various contributors seek to explore how knowledge and understanding may be learnt from reflection upon experience. Each contributor suggests that practice (indeed personal and social experience) is saturated with tacit theories and often unrecognized knowledge. These theories are at first only understandable if one is able to recognize the contexts and cultures (and the discourses that influence these) from which they emerge.

In Part 1 of Chapter 1, 'Psychosocial nursing: a model learnt from experience', my co-author, George Leach, and I give an overview of the emergence of psychosocial nursing over the last 50 years at the Cassel Hospital. Then, through a process of action research, we attempt to identify the beliefs and propositions that currently constitute psychosocial practice and the associated psychodynamic discourses which inform these. There is perhaps a tantalizing quality about the model of psychosocial practice they present, but the model is given substance and qualified meaning by the contributors in the next section, which highlights the use of such a model in practice.

Jacqueline Ord, in Chapter 2, considers the importance of subjective experience in social enquiry, and draws parallels between nursing practice and research methods which rely on direct observation. She illustrates the value of subjective data for nurses in the clinical setting, for people responsible for managing health care organizations, and for researchers.

Mimi Francis, in Chapter 3, considers the inevitability of change and transformation for us all at the level of individual experience but equally within the groups and institutions in which we live and work. She explores these themes through the implementation of a model of psychosocial practice at the Austen Riggs therapeutic community in the USA. She equally explores the need to understand and work with the distress caused within staff groups by the process of change and the importance of developing a systemic culture of understanding and collaboration.

Lastly, Gillian Chapman, in Chapter 4, explores the importance of discourse: the ideas, beliefs and theories which often invisibly shape and construct our experience. In particular, she considers what official government documents might say about the government policy of the day, and goes on to compare recent government care legislation with the principles of psychosocial practice.

Chapter 1
Psychosocial nursing: a model learnt from experience

Peter Griffiths and George Leach

Part 1

The Cassel Hospital: history and current practice

The Cassel Hospital for Functional Nervous Disorders was founded in 1921 by Sir Ernest Cassel. He had been impressed by the treatment of shell-shocked soldiers at Seale Hayne Military Hospital in Devon, after the First World War, and wished to endow a hospital for the treatment of civilians suffering from other functional nervous disorders. The first Medical Director, Dr T.A. Ross, had made a name for himself by successfully treating shell shock. He became interested in the psychological causes of neurosis, and this led to a more psychodynamic approach to therapy (Ross, 1923, 1932, 1936). In 1935, the first psychoanalyst (Clifford Scott) was appointed and patients received regular individual psychoanalysis. However, in other respects the hospital's social milieu reflected a more traditional hospital culture; nurses helped patients to meet their physical needs and managed the general domestic arrangements.

During the Second World War, the hospital was evacuated to Ash Hall near Stoke-on-Trent. The urgency of wartime involved both patients and staff being caught up in the war effort, turning their hands to working outside the institution. Having fewer trained personnel resulted in a decreased staff/patient ratio and this led to the introduction of group therapy and the extension of the nurses' and patients' roles into areas that were traditionally the province of other workers. A virtue was made of necessity and this trend continued in a more deliberate way after the war. As a consequence, the role of ancillary and paramedical staff was minimized.

The involvement of the patients in real work and the introduction of group therapy preceded the development of the hospital as a therapeutic community but, nevertheless, contributed towards its genesis.

After the Second World War, Dr Tom Main was appointed Medical Director. Together with the newly appointed Matron, Doreen Weddell, he was determined to develop the use of the hospital as a therapeutic institution, following experiments at Northfields Military Hospital during the war (Main, 1946; Ahrenfeldt, 1958; Bridger, 1985). By 1948, the orientation of the hospital was entirely psychoanalytical.

Main and Weddell went about developing the hospital as a therapeutic community (Barnes, 1968). Groups of nurses, doctors and patients met over a long period to examine the existing roles of patients and staff and their relevance to treatment and therapy (Main, 1967). As a consequence of these consultations, nursing practice gradually changed (Barnes, 1968) It adopted a less maternally nurturing and domesticated approach, and evolved into a form of nursing known as 'psychosocial nursing'.

Today, the hospital specializes in the inpatient treatment of individuals and whole families with severe emotional difficulties and problems. Most of the patients are admitted in a state of emotional and social breakdown. Physical and/or sexual abuse, deprivation and incidents of traumatic loss (of parents or of other members of the family), will often have been a feature of their past family backgrounds. Most of these patients have a long history of more conventional psychiatric treatment as either outpatients or inpatients. Depression, psychotic breakdown, overreliance on psychotropic medication and numerous episodes of self-harm and attempted suicide feature prominently in these histories.

Many of these patients have been diagnosed by referers as suffering from severe borderline or schizoid personality disorders. It is difficult to determine the extent to which the psychiatric profile of the patient group has changed since the founding of the hospital. External pressures and changing diagnostic practices and trends have had considerable influence.

Treatment comprises at least three interrelated aspects:

1. Individual psychoanalytical psychotherapy; in conjunction with this;
2. Psychosocial nursing (Barnes, 1968; Kennedy, et al., 1987; Griffith and Pringle, 1977) which takes place in the context of the therapeutic

community; and

3. Patients working actively and interacting with each other in the ordinary life of the community within the hospital.

The hospital's residential living and working environment forms the basis of a therapeutic milieu, and the framework within which nurses work with patients. Through the ongoing development and application of therapeutic community principles (Main, 1946; Barnes, 1968), the hospital has developed what it calls a 'culture of enquiry' (Main, 1983), which sets out actively to use the totality of the daily domestic and recreational aspects of living, in the service of the therapeutic work, so that the reasons for failures and successes in these everyday, but fundamentally important, situations can be explored and discussed.

Patients are expected to become active participants in the life and care of the hospital throughout their stay, sharing work, domestic and social activities, and joining with others (fellow patients and nurses). The hospital is socially structured around this living activity.

1. Patients take on real responsibilities for many everyday tasks as treatment progresses: cooking, cleaning and gardening. They graduate to elected positions of responsibility for managing the many groups that perform these kinds of activities.

2. All patients are supported by nursing staff; first, by a keyworker whom we call a 'primary nurse' (Weddell, 1968; Manthey, 1980). Secondly, in all their elected roles, they are partnered by a nurse. Every area of responsibility has a nurse manager working with a patient manager.

3. The whole of this elaborate system of activities is continuously scrutinized for its failings and successes by staff and patients. A system of meetings, overseen by a community management team, comprises two community meetings, unit meetings and various activities meetings, to report and receive observations on the running of the community and to discuss problems and ideas for improvement.

4. In parallel with this is a psychotherapeutic system, in which each primary nurse relates to a psychoanalytic psychotherapist, who will provide twice-weekly psychotherapy using individual or group methods.

The therapeutic community provides numerous arenas and different therapeutic milieux (de Lambert, 1982; James, 1987) for the exposure of the patient's neurotic difficulties. There is freedom and space for the patient's neurotic illnesses to be expressed and explored, and for the often chaotic, destructive behaviour, which the patient is driven to create and recreate, to be repeated in interactions with the patients and staff around them (Denford and Griffiths, 1993).

The hospital's daily life, with its variety of activities and relationships, allows opportunities for self-expression, experimentation and the testing out of previously acquired ways of relating to others and of doing things (van der Linden, 1988; Gabbard, 1992). This leads to reality testing, shared clarification, mutual learning, insight, change and growth.

Real responsibilities (and accountabilities) offer opportunities for both success and failure. The creation of a safe supportive environment, in which patients can experience failure and disappointment, as well as success, is an important part of the nursing work with these patients, in that it offers reparative possibilities. The development of pride in positive capacities and successes helps patients to cope with the inevitable pain in accruing insights into troubled areas of their personality.

> The hospital does not offer asylum as such, for the life of the community is often challenging and awkward, particularly for those individuals who tend to deny their own responsibility for their actions. Nonetheless it does offer patients a rare chance to face their difficulties within a therapeutic structure (Kennedy, 1987a: p. 1).

The development of psychosocial nursing

Since 1948, the Cassel has pioneered an action-based assessment and treatment model, integrating a practical use of psychoanalysis and social systems theory within a residential setting. This psychosocial treatment model involves a 'language' for understanding and practice in the use of actions and activity, as well as words and phantasies (Hinshelwood and Griffiths, 1987) (and their social representation). This model of thinking and practice has evolved and developed out of the often challenging and difficult work that the hospital undertakes with patients who present with severe emotional difficulties (Barnes, 1968).

The first formal training for nurses began in 1941, with an 18-month training for ward sisters who were interested in nursing patients with neurotic disturbances (Barnes, 1968).

In 1948, two kinds of training were offered: short intensive courses for nurses of various grades and from different fields of practice; and an 18-

month course for nurses of ward sister status. The former were run as summer schools and the latter at the hospital itself. The latter course evolved over a period of almost 50 years into an internally certificated course in psychological and family-centred nursing.

The intention of both courses was to feed back into the nursing profession the experience gained at the Cassel Hospital, in particular an understanding of patients as individuals and of their interactions within their families, within groups and as members of a larger hospital community.

In 1994, the 18-month course was redeveloped as a university-accredited two-year full-time Diploma in Psychosocial Nursing with Manchester University.

The practice of psychosocial nursing within this setting has also developed over time. These developments have occurred to meet changes in patients' needs, national developments in nursing practice, and the various restructurings of the National Health Service (Robinson, 1994). Most have occurred, however, through nurses themselves reflecting on their practice and on how it does or does not meet their, their patients' and the hospital's aspirations for care and treatment (Main, 1957; Barnes, 1968).

A good deal has been written about psychosocial nursing over the years; some of this has been published, but no explicit model has been described (Weddell, 1955; Barnes, 1968; Haque, 1973; Macklin, 1979; de Lambert, 1982; Chapman, 1984, 1988a, 1988b; Kennedy, 1987; Denford and Griffiths, 1993; Flynn, 1993; McCaffrey, 1994; Irwin, 1995).

Current psychosocial nursing practice

Nurses are based in one of the hospital's three units. Each has a case-load of patients. Wherever possible, the same nurse works with a patient throughout treatment. Nurses are responsible for making nursing assessments and devising treatment aims and plans with patients, to address their psychosocial problems. Nurses use psychosocial nursing principles to guide and inform their nursing practice within a therapeutic programme (Barnes, 1968; Chapman, 1984; Kennedy, 1987b).

The nurse attempts to form a relationship with the patient, within which, feelings, thoughts and ways of relating (by the patient to the nurse, as well as to others), can be talked about in as open and honest a way as possible in the here and now. The nurse uses his or her feelings and a personal sense of self as a therapeutic medium in relation to the patient (James, 1987), channelling transference and countertransference feelings into therapeutic responses.

In working alongside the patients in the day-to-day activities of community life, the nurse mediates between the physiological, psychological and social experiences of the patient through meaningful action and talk (Chapman, 1984; Flynn, 1993). Through reflection on this integrative process, the aim is to enable the patients to become more self-aware of their actions and aware of their effects on others, to develop a sense of responsibility for themselves and others, and to gain a real autonomy in their lives.

Within this overall structure, the nurses attempt to facilitate the patients' internal ego-functioning and their capacity to function at an everyday level within the various settings in the hospital, and to develop or reawaken motivation, creativity and initiative.

The nature of the attachment the patient forms with, or to, the primary nurse (as well as to other nurses and patients) provides a means for assessment. It also provides a means of exploration and possible reparation for the patient, as the patient moves from a way of relating based on previous earlier and later experience, to one based within the reality of the here and now (James, 1987).

The therapeutic programme is an interconnected structure of formal and informal meetings between staff and patients, doctors, therapists and nurses, both seniors and juniors. The patient's experience of the hospital, and others' experience (nurse, therapist and other patients) of the patient, are assessed and integrated within this structure of meetings.

Therapists attend a regular daily staff meeting with nurses and the therapeutic team to discuss an individual patient's progress, in an attempt to integrate information about the patient, derived from the various sources within the therapeutic milieu. The nurse–therapist relationship is monitored and supervised by more senior nurses and therapists in all these various settings. This provides not only a further guide to the patients' ways of relating (as these often reflect the nature of their parental and familial attachments) but also a way of understanding and making use of the complications that invariably arise within an inpatient psychotherapy setting (Main, 1957; Ploye, 1977; Hinshelwood, 1987; James, 1987).

The integration of these different aspects of treatment provides a structured predictable programme (James, 1987). In effect, this has a containing function in respect of the patient's projected aspects, as would an analytical session.

Part 2

Making explicit the Cassel model

Here, we describe a piece of action research, which was undertaken to identify and systematize the features of a model of psychosocial nursing practice. The derived model is set within the wider discourse about models of nursing practice and, particularly, the emerging debate about models of mental health practice.

Rationale

Many of the published papers concerning psychosocial nursing describe, in varying levels of detail, the process and practice of the Cassel model. However, any sense of a conceptual model that underpins and informs that practice has remained largely implicit within this literature and within the Cassel Hospital, its culture and its nurses. The reasons for this are speculative.

It is hard to make definitive statements about a model that is in a constant state of evolution and influenced by a variety of different professional discourses. It is, therefore, eclectic, and has, in effect, been hewn over the years. It is also a model that has been passed on implicitly through experience, through an oral and practical culture, as junior nurses learn from their more senior colleagues. Until now, the pressures or conditions have not existed to prompt anyone to define such a model in theoretical terms.

A kind of isolationism (that ended abruptly with the threat of hospital closure in 1990) made previous generations of nurses more inward looking and less interested in justifying the validity of their implicit model externally within the profession, and in disseminating the possibilities of its use elsewhere. Only more recently has there been a drive within the profession to work with models that originate from an academic approach. This demands nurses look at their practice at a more abstract level, rather than simply 'doing'. It is significant that nurses' initial and further education is now based within higher education establishments.

The Cassel Hospital Strategy for Nursing Group (a group of hospital nurses) identified the need to make explicit the psychosocial model of nursing practice, the treatment philosophy and the working practices in operation within the hospital. This need was also clearly identified by a marketing analysis undertaken by external consultants for the hospital at around the same time. A number of external and internal pressures dictated this need:

1. Our nursing practice assumptions were being sought and questioned, both internally by a variety of staff and externally by different agencies. An explicit psychosocial nursing model would help us to gain internal and external clarity (with health care purchasers, for example).

2. A model of psychosocial nursing was needed for there to be a grounded, rational, future development of nursing and nursing practice, whether this was to be within the hospital's inpatient services or outside, either in different health care settings or the community.

3. A psychosocial nursing model was desirable for the redevelopment and accreditation of the psychosocial nursing course. It was also important for the development of coherent learning objectives that were applicable to the course.

4. A model would provide a framework for teaching within the hospital, for use by other staff and course nurses (as an agreed frame of reference) and for use in external training, either for formal teaching or for use in consultancy work with other organisations.

5. A model was needed to underpin a shared frame of reference for ongoing nursing practice: to help with the formulation of nursing aims, the identification of outcomes for practice, and report writing, for example. It would also provide a more coherent means by which these might be assessed and worked with under supervision.

6. A model would provide a baseline for future research in psychosocial nursing, and make a comparison with other models possible.

7. A model might well help other professional groups (child and adult psychotherapists) and professionals on placement within the hospital better to understand nursing practice within the therapeutic milieu.

8. It was also felt that a model of psychosocial nursing made explicit, identified with and *owned by the nursing staff of the hospital*, would provide a clearer rationale for working practice and offer something that could be criticized and reworked. It might also promote a greater autonomy and effectiveness in practice, as well as a greater integration with the various working practices within the hospital.

Main (1989) had suggested many years earlier that any health-seeking system must be self-monitoring, exploratory of its relations, and capable of self-modification. He suggested that the hallmark of this was not a particular form of social structure but a sustained *culture of enquiry* into its personal, interpersonal and intersystem relationships and their strengths, weaknesses and difficulties. The present authors felt that, whilst this approach had continued to inform the hospital's work with patients in promoting insight, growth and development, its use had declined in rigour as a method of enquiry by staff into their own practice. It seemed that the hospital's culture (and this included the nursing culture) had gradually accepted, unthinkingly, the ideas and rationales handed down from one generation to the next. Ideas had moved from the experimental and thinking areas of the ego of one generation into the fixed-morality areas, the ego ideal and the superego, of the next (Main, 1967).

The explicit, alive, thought-through rationales for practice, and reasons for action or nonaction, became implicit or forgotten. What had replaced them, or developed instead, were sometimes ritualized, hollow practices. The hospital's strengths and weaknesses in terms of its therapeutic rationale (and nursing rationales) had become implicit and increasingly rarified. It was, therefore, felt that the identification of an explicit working model might encourage and allow for a living discourse of ideas around our practice and a demystification of the historical cultural assumptions about Cassel nursing.

It is also a model of practice which the authors believe can be adapted and applied to a variety of health care settings (hence this book), but perhaps especially within the field of mental health care provision.

Psychosocial practice in other settings

The prevalence of personality disorders is difficult to determine, but one study identified such disorders in 13 percent of an urban population (Casey and Tyrer, 1986). Tyrer et al. (1993) note that 'recent inquiries into the prevalence and type of personality disorders in psychiatric inpatients have shown that nearly half qualify for the diagnosis', and conclude that 'personality disorder is a ubiquitous companion to psychiatric practice' (p. 10). This chronic and disabling mental illness typically presents as self-mutilation, suicidal behaviour, inappropriate aggression and incapacitating neuroses, low self-esteem, depression, and inappropriate or absent social relationships. Spontaneous remission for these patients is very rare and, without appropriate treatment, many of them will kill themselves or deteriorate to the point of irreversible helplessness. Numerous studies have shown that these patients are a significant drain on NHS resources through repeated attendance at general practitioners' surgeries and accident and emergency departments, numerous stays in inpatient and visits to outpatient psychiatric departments, and through repeated prescription costs. Often, the only possibility of effective treatment is through inpatient care in specialized psychotherapeutic units (Rosser, et al. 1987; Dolan, et al. 1992; Chiesa, et al. 1996). This evident need has not been matched by a sufficient level of research, professional education, or treatment provision. The Cassel Hospital has developed a model of treatment and practice for working with people with borderline personality disorder and the psychosocial model of nursing practice is a major part of that model.

With the advent of 'care in the community' for the mentally ill, as a result of the National Health Service and Community Act, 1990, there has been a proliferation of small units of mental health workers providing mental health care within residential and day care settings. While there is a variety of different practice and management models in operation, the two are rarely linked into one coherent model. Moreover, there is an absence of any theoretically integrated clinical model that underpins both practice and clinical management. This results in a provision of care and treatment which is often inconsistent and equally frustrating for patients and staff. The therapeutic potential of the environmental context, the social milieu and the person, is rarely realized, leading often to a sense of failure. We believe the Cassel model of psychosocial practice, if made explicit, can be used in these settings.

Nursing models

Of models in nursing, Fawcett (1984: p. 3) states:

> The utility of conceptual models comes from the organization they provide for thinking, for observations and for interpreting what is seen. Conceptual models also provide a systematic structure and a rationale for activities. Furthermore they give direction to the search for relevant questions about phenomena and they point out solutions to practical problems. Conceptual models also provide criteria for knowing when a problem has been solved.

Fawcett (1984: p. 4) however, also acknowledges: 'A model is, however, only an approximation or simplification of reality, a representation of the world that includes only those concepts that the model builder considers relevant.'

This statement reflects a view that nursing models have tended to be based on value judgements and reflect the bias and interests of the model builder. This has resulted in a disparity between the model-makers and the model-users – the practitioners of nursing.

Nursing models produced in earlier years by academic nursing theorists, were mainly produced by those working in the USA and mainly related to general nursing. This burgeoning model-making process has been criticized, and some have questioned whether models of nursing are necessary. In order to justify the introduction and elaboration of yet another model, it is necessary to review these criticisms so that a context can be established.

Kenny (1993) asserts that there are several common reasons why nursing models have failed in practice. The fact that they are derived from or invented by academics and then applied by nurse managers and educationalists in a 'top-down' way, makes it hard for individual practitioners to gain a sense of value and utility and to recognize the language and values of a particular model as being in accordance with their own.

Nurses' sense of alienation may lead to resistance, provoking academic misunderstanding at the perceived failure of nurses to adopt models with sufficient imagination and enthusiasm. Those who comment on practice are not always those who are doing it, which is a trend that is set to continue with the wholesale removal of nurse education in the United Kingdom into the higher education arena and away from an apprenticeship system.

Too often, models have been introduced with a lack of appropriate educational preparation and in-service training. This creates difficulties which may be compounded during the implementation phase if there is a lack of necessary support, especially if new jargon has to be learned and there has to be adjustment to new (and additional) paperwork.

Nurses' scepticism may be compounded by a feeling that the introduction of a particular model may be a passing fad, rather than the foundation for a long-lasting change in practice. Such new models are not introduced into a vacuum and, therefore, may run counter to deeply cherished assumptions held by nurses, and counter to expectations of other professionals, potentially leading to interdisciplinary conflict.

Such models may be imposed on an unwilling group of patients; for example Kenny (1993) points out that the concept of self-responsibility (Orem, 1980) is not necessarily seen as a desirable aim of treatment by all patients, certainly not by those with particular struggles with dependency, as might be found at the Cassel Hospital. The vast majority of nursing models have originated in the USA, and most of these depict nursing as a rational, problem-solving, practical process (i.e. the 'nursing process'). Lundh, et al. (1988) have expressed, from a European perspective, their reservations about this American dominance. Nursing is not purely based on reasoning but is informed and influenced by conscious and unconscious cultural bias. The nursing process can objectify and put an unhelpful distance between the patient and the nurse by being based on normative and positivist assumptions about standards of behaviour.

Foucault (1965, 1973, 1987) suggests that medical, psychiatric and psychoanalytical discourse is characterized by a preoccupation with surveillance, definition and control of patients' internal psychic and external domestic and bodily functions. Rose (1985, 1989) has powerfully developed this line of thinking further, suggesting that a range of technologies of subjectivity have been developed and that these discourses shape and enhance the psychological capacities of citizens in many latent ways.

Hiraki (1992) (see also Chapman, 1988a, 1988b) in an analysis of the language of nursing textbooks, questions the uncritical acceptance of the 'nursing process' as a rational scientific activity. She questions whether nursing is properly seen as a problem-solving activity, as an activity that is empirically based and, therefore, free of values. Further, Habermas and McCarthy (1976) felt that an understanding of the political dimensions of labour and power was also necessary, fully to understand social action.

Nurses perhaps gain respectability by being scientific. Will this, paradoxically, gain them independence from medicine, or provide a pyrrhic victory where status is apparently won, but where nurses are confirmed in a subservient role to medicine (i.e. an ancillary 'profession')? The danger of political and economic considerations being excluded is that core nursing qualities and values, such as interpersonal communication, cultivated intuition, compassion, trust and altruism, will be presented as mere 'skills', in a way that empties them of their true meaning and power.

The fact that nurses have implemented models in an ambivalent and piecemeal way illustrates something important, or even essential, about the relationship between nursing practice and theory: that nurses themselves and the nurse–patient relationship should be participants in the theoretical discourse, not simply the passive recipients of its attention (Sheehan, 1996).

Just as most models relate to general nursing, the critique of nursing models has largely ignored mental health nursing. Indeed, the problems are perhaps even greater in the mental health field because aspects of models are borrowed from general nursing and from other disciplines. Clarke (1988) suggests that nursing models used in mental health are generally untested, rely heavily on humanistic assumptions (General Nursing Council for England and Wales, 1982) and are perhaps a politically convenient alternative to the medical model. They, however, expose the nurse to potential conflict and eventual disillusionment because of the political realities of ward life; the medical model prevails, and the patients themselves are an unco-operative disappointment, seemingly impervious to humanistic interventions by nurses, laden with unconditional positive regard, warmth and empathy. While other theoretical approaches are available to mental health nurses, the work at the Cassel Hospital is most easily understood from a psychoanalytical frame of reference.

Psychodynamic models of nursing

The use and application of psychoanalytical ideas within nursing practice has a chequered history. Over the years, various groups of interested nurses have established groups to further the utilization of psychoanalytical ideas within nursing practice. Several hospitals have run the English National Board for Nursing Course 660, Psychodynamic Techniques for Nurses. The Nurses' Association for Psychodynamic Psychotherapy was established in the 1980s to secure the right of nurses to practise psychotherapy within the NHS. The Royal College of Nursing had, for a while, a Psychodynamic Education Group and ran a certificated therapeutic communities course in association with the Association of Therapeutic Communities. Neither of these exist any longer.

In 1990, the Association for Psychoanalytic Psychotherapy in the NHS (APP) ran a conference entitled 'Ethics and Emotions in Nursing', and, while the conference was poorly attended, a number of fascinating papers was published identifying the usefulness and relevance of psychoanalytical thinking to the understanding and application of nursing practice (Conran, 1991; Fabricius, 1991; Goldie, 1991; Wright, 1991). More recently, the APP has established a nursing subdivision. This organizes regular seminars that explore the application of psychoanalytical and psychodynamic ideas to nursing practice, as well as an annual conference. Yet, at the time of writing, it might be appropriate to concur with Winship (1995: p. 289), in his review of the relationship between nursing and psychoanalysis, when he suggests: 'The relationship between psychoanalysis and nursing is still far from well defined, and for the most part, psychoanalytic ideas are perceived with some antipathy by the majority of nurses'.

The most well-known application of psychoanalytical thinking to nursing practice is perhaps contained within Hildegard Peplau's work on nursing. Following her work at Chestnut Lodge (an inpatient psycho-therapy unit in the USA) and under the influence of Erica Fromm and Harry Stack-Sullivan, Peplau developed and advocated a psychoanalytical approach to nurses' work with psychiatric patients (Peplau, 1952). She reiterated this approach more recently when she suggested that psychi-atric nurses should include 50-minute, scheduled talking 'sessions' with their patients on three days a week (Peplau, 1994: p. 5). It is important to note that this approach involves nurses adopting an additional profession, psychoanalytical psychotherapy, rather than continuing to be nurses. However, as Winship (1995: p. 295) points out, Peplau maintained then and now that: 'It is the nurse herself who is the agent of change for a patient rather than the mechanism or the type of therapy.'

Peplau's model has been influential in mental health nursing theory, but perhaps less so in practice. It is an eclectic model, inductively derived and influenced by theorists external to nursing. The nurse is seen as having an educative, therapeutic and maturing (nurturing) role, a sort of counselling educator who somehow deals with and resolves complex interpersonal issues (such as transference) along the way. However, with a heavy emphasis on dyadic psychodynamics (the dyad of nurse and patient), Peplau undervalues and underdevelops the psychosocial and sociocultural dimensions of the patient's human condition.

While these ideas took root in the USA, and to some extent influenced philosophically the content of postgraduate mental health nurse training there, an explicit psychoanalytically informed model of mental health nursing (rather than one that amounts to nurses becoming psychotherapists) has not been attempted. In the UK, the influence of psychoanalytical ideas on the nursing profession as a whole has been comparatively weak, occurring mainly within therapeutic communities (Hinshelwood and Manning, 1979), at a few other sites (Hughes and Halek, 1991), and at the Maudsley Hospital, London (Jackson and Cawley, 1992; Jackson and Williams, 1994).

Peplau's attempts at Chestnut Lodge to co-operate in an alliance between the nursing and psychoanalytical professions were rebuffed, which prompted her to develop her own model. In contrast, Doreen Weddell, matron of the Cassel Hospital in Tom Main's time, enjoyed a more co-operative relationship, but one which perhaps paradoxically led to psychosocial nursing occupying a position in the academic background (or backwater?). This was never made explicit as a model, but it was implicit within the nursing work that developed under her leadership.

Tom Main, (in an unpublished address, 'On the history of the Cassel Hospital', given in 1976 to the hospital's Jubilee Conference) had clear views on this and indeed on the undesirability of nurses working to a professional model:

> . . . I ceased to hope that nursing would become a profession and hoped that it would remain a craft, a matter of skill rather than scholarship, and set about thinking together with the Matron of ways we could help them become less

apologetic about lack of scholarship and more sure about their care functions.

Indeed, Main saw the desire of nurses to involve themselves in scholarship as being defensive in nature:

> The strains of caring for severely neurotic people are many and some of the nurses sought various defences against contact with the patients' suffering – more scholarship, more lectures, more distancing, more contact with doctors . . .

If psychosocial nursing is to be known, understood and applied in other settings, however, the implicit must be made explicit. Inevitably, this means that the underlying principles and practice of a discoverable model take on a new existence, as nursing theory. This seems to contradict Tom Main's views, which, in any case, could have been influenced by the prevailing cultural attitudes and assumptions about women, women's work and their place in the professions and society. Yet, he was also drawing attention to the need to develop understanding and knowledge through practice. The model described here does not set out to reject entirely the notion of apprenticeship in nursing, but supports its integration with theory.

Indeed, an increasingly accepted view in modern nursing theory (Benner, 1984; Draper, 1992; Lacey, 1993) is that embedded theory should be derived from practice, that models should be discovered rather than invented, and that tools developed from practice theories will have a high degree of utility and, therefore, be less likely to be regarded as dogma, than tools born of an idealized vision of nursing, imposed on an unwilling workforce.

Clarke (1988: p. 13), too, says that change will hardly come about by fashionable literary attempts to present nursing in a way that nurses find unrecognizable. In mental health there has been a dearth of descriptive studies, few on ideology and few on attitudes. This produces cynicism and apathy because there is a lack of perspective to guide them, a lack of recognition of the value of apprenticeship caused by a split between theory and the real world.

The model of psychosocial nursing that we describe here aims to be a living, comprehensive, reflexive and, therefore, valid model that involves both nurses and patients in its continuing evolution.

Research design: action research

It would have been possible for us theoretically to have constructed a speculative or deductive account or model of what psychosocial nursing is, without undertaking any active research, drawing on our own knowledge base as practitioners. However (in order to define the current operational model of psychosocial nursing), it seemed important to work collaboratively with the hospital's nurses and patients, to reveal the tacit assumptions that underpinned current psychosocial practice.

'Co-operative enquiry' is an overall term used to describe the various approaches to research *with* people, as opposed to research *on* people. We would argue, like Reason (1988: p.4), that: 'Orthodox research methods are inadequate for a science of persons, quite simply because they undermine the self determination of their subjects.' He argues that what, above all, distinguishes humanity is people's ability to choose how they will act and the capacity to give meaning to their experience and to their actions:

> Orthodox scientific method (particularly the formal experiment, but following this surveys, questionnaires, and observation) aims quite systematically and intentionally to exclude the subjects from all choice about the subject matter of the research, all consideration of appropriate inquiry method, all the creative thinking that goes into making sense of it; and it therefore excludes from the field of research just that aspect of being self determination – which particularly characterizes the subjects as persons.

Co-operative enquiry seeks knowledge in action and for action. It places an emphasis on participation and wholeness. It is not interested in either fragmented knowing, or theoretical knowing that is separated from practice and experience. As a method, it seeks a knowing-in-action which encompasses as much of the participants' experience as possible.

Holter and Schwartz-Barcot (1993: p. 302) have described this approach to research under the rubric of 'action research'. The method adopted here perhaps exemplifies the type of action research that they term the 'enhancement approach'. They suggest in this approach that:

> The researcher raises questions about the underlying assumptions and values and involves the practitioners in critically reflecting on their practice and bringing to light the difference between stated practices, underlying assumptions and unwritten laws which really govern that practice. The researcher facilitates the practitioners' discussion of underlying problems and assumptions on a personal level as well as the level of the organisation's culture and the possible conflicts they can generate . . . Local theory emerges from reflective discussions between the researcher and practitioner.

This method of research enquiry was appropriate to our work for a number of reasons. We hoped it would retain a sensitivity to social processes, while encouraging those involved in the enquiry to participate as co-researchers and to identify their own and the organization's learning and developmental needs. It was also a method well suited to liberating social actors from overprescribed institutional role-play. Significantly, as a method of research it was not so far removed from that of a therapeutic community's practice. It allowed for an evaluation and creative critique of social phenomena, drawing on the experiential fabric of the community and its practices to this end.

Manning (1979), in discussing the outcome of Rapoport's (1960) research work at the Henderson Hospital, suggests that, unless research in this field can become a joint participative exercise, whereby problems that the community wishes to resolve can be tackled (but without a naive faith that the solution, which, if it can be found, will come easily) it tends to be either ignored and rejected, or treated as a kind of magic.

The research process needs not only to be sanctioned but participative ownership by those involved in the project and any subsequent developments commenced. Towell and Harries (1979) have suggested that any attempt to cut short the work of change by directly imposing new practices, or grafting new practices on top of old ones, inadequately recognizes the significance of each staff group having to engage in the process of innovation. Greenwood (1984) suggests that clinical nurses and researchers together need to decide on the identification and diagnosis of a problem and plan the action to correct it because the clinical nurses themselves are the ones who, directly or indirectly, implement any plans for development or change.

Research methodology

All the nurses within the Cassel Hospital were provided with written information, explaining the project and its rationale. This research initiative was discussed in a variety of nursing settings within the hospital, seeking the nurses' participation in the venture.

A series of workshops was arranged to take place over a number of months. Each was attended by all of the members of a particular grade of the nursing staff (i.e. 'F' grade nurses attended one, 'G' grade nurses another, 'H' grade nurses and the Lead Nurse another). A group of patients took part in the last workshop.

The rationale for splitting the grades and workshops was that the possibility of working with the whole nurse group at any one time would have been pragmatically unfeasible and group-dynamically unmanageable. Some grades of nurse might have been influenced by their managers and supervisors being present. In addition, it would not have been possible to determine whether different grades held different opinions and rationales about the nature of nursing in the hospital.

As it turned out, there was a considerable degree of consistency across the grades about the nature of psychosocial nursing. The differences lay in the areas of nursing focus and the sophistication of the language with which it was described.

In each workshop, the same format was followed and the groups were invited to brainstorm each of the following questions:

1. What are the philosophical beliefs and values that inform psychosocial nursing at the Cassel Hospital?
2. What are the intended outcomes and goals of psychosocial nursing for both the practitioner and the patient/s?
3. What are the principles involved in the process of nursing that aim to achieve these goals?
4. What knowledge, skills and attitudes do nurses need in order to participate in this process?

These questions follow the format originated by Pearson and Vaughan (1986) and seemed a readily useful framework to use. One of us scribed the answers while the other facilitated the process by drawing out nuances and clarifying oft-quoted 'Casselisms' (nursing clichés and stock phrases such as 'work alongside' and 'take responsibility for'), helping the participant and the group to unpack what such phrases might mean to them. It was also important to use language that would be understood outside the hospital.

It was agreed that notes of the sessions would be written up from the material produced and circulated to the respective nurse groups to check for accuracy and to note any comments, reflections and further thoughts. It was also agreed to collate all the material from the four workshops and try to derive a model of psychosocial nursing which might then either be circulated and/or presented at a nurses' forum (a regular internal arena for discussion).

Analysis: the model

By asking groups of nurses to brainstorm their responses to the four questions, it was intended to elicit their views on psychosocial nursing's philosophy, goals and objectives, principles, practice, it's body of knowledge, skills and attitudes. A very large amount of data resulted, which was analysed in relation to Fawcett's (1984) four central concepts, which underlie the metaparadigm of nursing, according to nursing theorists, and, therefore, are embedded within all valid nursing models.

> Considerable agreement now exists that the central concepts of the discipline of nursing are: person, environment, health and nursing. Person refers to the recipient of nursing actions who may be an individual, a family, a community, or a particular group. Environment refers to the recipient's significant others

and surroundings, as well as to the setting in which nursing actions occur. Health refers to the wellness and/or illness state of the recipient. And, nursing refers to the actions taken up by nurses on behalf of or in conjunction with the recipient (Fawcett, 1984: p. 6).

It was felt to be important that the model should meet Fawcett's requirements. By categorizing the results of the research, integrating Pearson's and Vaughan's (1986) format within Fawcett's four concepts, the intention was to analyse and make explicit the Cassel psychosocial nursing model. Following Fawcett, the model is presented in the form of abstract and general beliefs, concepts and propositions. Where relevant, reference is made to appropiate work written about the hospital that further illustrate these concepts, and to the psychoanalytical and systems theories (and theorists) used in the nursing lecture programme at the hospital. These metatheories and ideas underpin and inform many of the propositions made.

Figure 1.1 illustrates the structure of the psychosocial model of practice. There are four main components, which relate to Fawcett's (1984) metaparadigms:

Environment   Person   Health   Nursing

Within each of these metaparadigms the following four central concepts are explored (see tables on pages 24–31):

- Philosophy of psychosocial nursing;
- Goals and outcomes of psychosocial nursing (for practitioner and patient);
- Principles intended to achieve the goals, outcomes of psychosocial nursing;
- Nurses', knowledge, skills and attitudes.

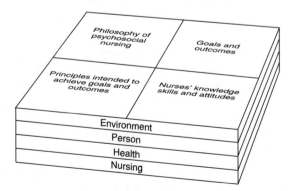

Figure 1.1   A psychosocial model of practice.

Table 1.1

Environment

Philosophy

Shared endeavour and responsibility can produce more than individual effort alone, and create a reality-oriented matrix for growth. By creating a specialized environment for treatment that reflects many aspects of the external world, yet allows greater permissiveness, difficulties and psychological disturbance can emerge and be detected because of the distortions that occur in structures, roles, responsibilities and communication. If these disturbances can be contained mentally by nurses, through a process of reflection, and understood (rather than medicated), it is possible to create a therapeutic 'culture of enquiry'. Of this culture, Main (1989: p. 141) suggested:

> The hallmark of such an organisation was not a particular form of social structure but a culture of enquiry. It both requires and sanctions instruments of enquiry into personal and interpersonal and inter-system problems, the study of impulses, defences and relations as these are expressed and arranged socially.

The whole treatment environment, and the boundary between it and aspects of the external environment, with the rich array of everyday events they provide, have the potential to be used in this way (Kennedy, 1987).

The emerging disturbance will to some extent be a re-enactment of past experiences (by an individual, couple, family, group or community). Psychic and behavioural change may be possible through a registering of re-enactment, working through, understanding and reconstruction of thoughts, feelings and acts (James, 1987: p. 82). Reconstruction is possible with:

* Clear rules and boundaries;
* Tolerance and understanding of group and individual freedoms, rights and responsibilities;
* Mutual respect and directness;
* A degree of certainty and safety which holds the patient's level of anxiety to a level which is possible to tolerate.

It is important to keep all channels of communication open (or to examine the distortions that emerge) in order to maintain the therapeutic quality of the environment.

Goals and outcomes

The environment needs to be reliable, stable and safe enough to allow for experimentation with some success and survivable failure, in a climate of mutual trust. Events that happen within such an environment cease to be random, but they can be monitored in a systematic manner and seen as meaningful. An overcontrolled or chaotic environment cannot be used as a therapeutic milieu (James and Wilson, 1987).

Principles intended to achieve the goals and outcomes

The physical and social environment needs to be psychologically robust enough for strong feelings to be expressed, recognized, explored and contained. The environment provides a sufficiently permissive climate in which challenging behaviour and feelings can be expressed, but, equally and in turn, challenged by collective and mutual enquiry (Morrice, 1979).

Time is important in the therapeutic environment. There are reliable, consistent and reality-oriented sequences of events, which provide a 24-hour managed framework for the life of the hospital. Individual or social disturbance can be monitored when these time boundaries are transgressed or distorted, and the meaning of this explored.

Time and structured events interrelate to generate expectations of behaviour and participation. These are more fully and formally expressed in the provision of opportunities for real responsibility and reality-oriented work, in the form of specific roles and jobs and how they are taken up and performed (Bion, 1961; Kennedy, 1987; Menzies-Lyth, 1989b).

Knowledge, skills and attitudes

Nurses need a knowledge base and related skills that are sufficient to create and maintain a safe and therapeutic physical and social environment: health and safety, food hygiene, and the establishment of expectations in community living. The exercise of these skills brings the nurse into contact with the environment and its wider therapeutic potential.

Table 1.2

Person

Philosophy

On entering the hospital, people do not lose their human and civil rights, and should have their individuality and an understanding of those rights respected, provided they do not compromise the rights of others. Children have rights too and these should not be subordinated to their parents' or other adults' needs.

It is important to develop a collaborative understanding with the whole person, not merely a relationship with the presenting symptoms, difficulties or underlying pathology. Every person has a mixture of functioning and nonfunctioning parts, aspects, strengths and weaknesses, both internally and in their relationship with the psychosocial environment. Therefore, everyone has something to offer and something to gain (nurses and patients alike) in the development of reciprocal and reflexive relationships. People have resources and capacities that can be further developed if those individuals have the desire and motivation to change.

Freud's (1966) maxim representing the fundamental goals of the human condition, 'to love and to work', should inform nursing work, much of which is aimed at improving self-esteem, interpersonal relationships and generativity, through the relationships which can emerge out of work activity (Jaques, 1960).

Goals and outcomes

The creation and provision of 'good enough' (Winnicott, 1965) and safe enough relationships (patient–patient, patient–nurse, parent–child, nurse–nurse, and so on) are required for the nurturing of personal identity and growth and the containing of individual and group disturbance. An increased sense of self-awareness and self-worth within an individual can be developed within the interpersonal matrix of these relationships. This enables the individuals to acquire an increased sense of responsibility for their behaviour and its effect on others. It also permits a sense of achievement that accrues from participation in the daily life of the hospital community. It can lead to the development of sufficient trust in self and others, to sustain people in more productive and fulfilled lives outside.

The continued use of supportive services outside the hospital follows a pattern of healthy dependency, rather than the inappropriate, wasteful and self-defeating pattern that existed before admission (Oldman, 1995; Chiesa, et al. 1996). In the continued development of the family unit, parents and children have equal opportunity for age-appropriate growth.

Principles intended to achieve the goals and outcomes.

The minimum requirements are:

- An ability to engage with the environment provided, to the extent that people can take on some responsibility for themselves and others;
- A belief in the capacity for change that can be initiated through partnership and shared ownership of the therapeutic process and environment. An expectation of participation in, and shared ownership of, the capacity for change;
- An ability to work on personal difficulties within individual(one-to-one) and group settings so that joint exploration, planning and review can help to define and expedite individual and family goals;
- Having and holding on to a home outside of the hospital to lessen institutionalization and ensure that real social issues can be worked on and brought into the treatment setting;
- Engagement with the therapeutic programme needs to be recognized ultimately as an engagement not based on the pursuit of efficiency, but on the realization of therapeutic potential.

Knowledge, skills and attitudes

Nurses value and create opportunities for the revelation of knowledge about the person, the patient, the parent–child relationship and the family (in the expression of their unique identity) in diverse situations, over time. This leads to an authentic, unfolding sense of identity and of the difficulties the patient may be experiencing in life, rather than a sterile gathering of historical data, from which speculative hypotheses are created.

Patients can also be understood through the nurse's countertransference. The feelings about and experiences of the patient in relation to the nurse, others and the environment, if registered and used, deepen and enhance the patient's sense of identity and others' knowledge of them (Chapman, 1984; James, 1987; Denford and Griffiths, 1993). Nurses need to foster in patients the ability to maintain hope (Denford and Griffiths, 1993) and to equip themselves with strategies that will maximize their sense of fulfilment and a positive attitude about themselves. Nurses also need to foster an attitude in patients that favours the engagement in words rather than in self-destructive deeds. It is also important, however, to note that deeds often have a symbolic meaning, which can be recovered through words. It is important for nurses to convey knowledge about external resources in relation to employment, education and housing, and to deploy this in the most appropriate way, to enable the patient to make best use of it.

Success is not all. Failing and failures can be made use of and learned from if held to be valuable experiences.

Table 1.3

Health

Philosophy

An individual's physical and mental systems are multidimensional interrelated states, forming a holistic system. Different parts of that system can be relatively healthy or unhealthy at any one time and are experienced as such to varying degrees by that person and by other people. Neither health nor illness are absolute states but are socially constructed and defined by and through an interaction between internal and externally derived factors.

Dependency evolves over the lifespan, taking different forms, and is an essential feature of humans as individual and social beings. It is not, as some nursing models portray it (for example: Orem, 1980) simply an undesirable regressive state to be combated and ultimately eradicated by health care professionals. Human development is a lifelong holistic process, the components of which can stay constant, stagnate, regress or evolve over time (Rayner, 1986).

Goals and outcomes

Surviving suicidal and self-destructive feelings is a prerequisite to the achievement of any further goals (Hale and Campbell, 1991).

If the range and depth of biopsychosocial areas of functioning are increased, reflective learning leads to increased self-awareness, sensitivity, and the ability to examine and understand the origins of ideas and feelings. Emotional capacity, social and daily living skills, and adaptability, are also increased.

Health goals need to be orientated to social reality and to facilitate an increased awareness of choices and resources and the ability to make use of them, and an increased capacity to negotiate and work with conflict, and to take developmental risks and experiment.

It takes courage to be authentic (true to oneself and others) while continuing to function in the face of distress or difficulties, but this can lead to an increase in mature dependency, individuation, and an increased use of human relationships rather than the use of statutory services.

Principles intended to achieve the goals and outcomes

Mental health and mental illness are not in a linear relationship in simple opposition to each other, but can be thought of as two separate continua (Trent, 1992) or axes (Downie, 1990).

Psychosocial nursing seeks actively to promote mental health, which to some extent will alleviate the types of mental illness encountered or treated at the Cassel Hospital. Mental illness is viewed in terms of the 'continuous' explanatory model of psychoanalysis, which has a less dichotomous basis than psychiatry, which is a discontinuous model that clearly separates those defined as mentally ill and those who are mentally healthy (Siegler and Osmond, 1976).

Psychosocial nursing also promotes: the capacity of the individual; the group and the social environment to interact in ways that promote a sense of well-being; the optimal development and use of mental abilities (thinking, feeling and relating); and the achievement of individual and collective goals, in a way that is consistent with justice and equality.

Knowledge, skills and attitudes

Nurses evolve a concept of, and a body of, knowledge about health as a normative social construct that needs to be engaged in with patients, rather than as an absolute or idealized category. Nurses develop skills to highlight the connected effect of a patient's relationship with his or her own health, on his or her social relationships.

Table 1.4

Nursing

Philosophy

Nurses need to develop a strong internal sense of their role and responsibility, if they are to maintain a therapeutic presence that will enable them to detect disturbance elsewhere within the psychosocial system (Main, 1989).

The potential for change can be more fully realized if the nurse believes in the existence and value of a psychosocial dimension to care, rather than seeing the provision of care as a one-to-one curative act, determined by the performance of a particular skill or intervention performed by the 'active nurse' upon the 'passive patient' (Main, 1975). An individual's best hope for change may instead be located within and held singularly, or in a combination of the physical, psychological or social domains, at an individual, interpersonal, group or community level.

Nurses can hold on to hope and hopefulness if they can own and contain their own omnipotent phantasies of absolute cure and its converse – total impotence or failure – and recognize that the possibility of change resides in the psychosocial matrix (Meinrath and Roberts, 1982; Dartington, 1994; Roberts, 1994).

Goals and outcomes

The goals and objectives of nursing should be congruent with those associated with health, the person and the environment, so that, for nurses, personal and professional development are closely related and interdependent.

Psychosocial nursing is more than goal- and outcome-oriented. It is a process aimed at the provision of 'good enough' (Winnicott, 1965) nurture and caring, which provides the matrix for possible transformation, rather than omnipotently seeking to cure a symptom or disease.

Principles intended to achieve the goals and outcomes

Although some need for dependency in patients is recognized (and this may vary over time), nurses strive to work with patients towards a sharing of responsibility for care and the outcome of treatment.

This complex, and by no means straightforward, process forms the basis of the nurse–patient relationship. Similarities and differences between the respective roles of nurse and patient are not denied but acknowledged and form the basis for a potential collaborative alliance for work with the patient. This alliance also allows for conflict, which is inevitable because of differing responsibilities, roles, expectations and levels of mutual identification and understanding. There is a recognition that these processes are going on in parallel, within a network of relationships throughout the hospital community. Staff and patient identification of these patterns of relatedness plays a role in both assessment and treatment and is one of the important ways in which the group is used to support the individual (nurse and patient) in the pursuit of understanding.

A truly collaborative relationship (nurse–patient or patient–patient) that avoids collusion, yet allows for and makes use of conflict, is a real relationship, dependent on the appropriate (with a professional focus) spontaneous and authentic use of self and feelings, rather than the stereotyped and defensive use of a professional persona (Menzies, 1960; Tonnesman, 1979; Roberts, 1994).

Nurses utilize their awareness of self and associated thoughts and feelings in the here and now in their engagement with patients. They also use a psychodynamic frame of reference to explore with the patient how previous experiences and events may be impinging on their present relationships. This is a nursing use of transference and its corollary, countertransference (Salzberger-Wittenberg, 1970; Schroder, 1985; James 1987).

The potential for creative change is located within this network of relationships, rather than in a dependence on external agents, such as medication or substance use, or in dysfunctional relationships. Sometimes, a high degree of continuity, consistency and perseverance will be necessary for such change to be realized.

Nurses working in this way offer both a model and catalyst to other nurses and patients, the aim of which is to be both empathic and yet challenging about the potential for change (Morrice, 1979). This type of work is made possible by a particular use of boundaries which demarcate particular areas of social experience and expectation. They provide a container, in Bion's (1970) sense, for psychological disturbance, and as described in terms of the therapeutic community by Hinshelwood (1987). They can be used in the service of systemic awareness, rather than simply as rules of conduct or as defensive rituals (Menzies, 1960). Vicissitudes within such a system are informative about the disturbance that creates it, and maybe enquired into. Similarly, vicissitudes within the multidisciplinary team, inside and outside the hospital, may resonate with the patients' disturbance and vice versa (Stanton and Schwartz, 1954; Main, 1957).

Predictable everyday structures, such as cleaning, cooking, play groups and social activities, provide a reality (both external and internal) which can be engaged with and managed by both nurses and patients (Rapoport, 1960; Flynn, 1993; Irwin, 1995). The need to break down global and potentially overwhelming tasks into more manageable ones serves both an intrapsychic and a social need. At an intrapsychic level, real responsibilities and associated activities provide a medium for an exploration of issues such as omnipotence, guilt (blame and shame), and despair, as well as reparation (Klein, 1975). At the social level, it helps to subdivide the project of cooking a meal for 60 people into achievable subtasks. This also has the effect of challenging the view that all relationships are destructive.

Stress and strain are conventionally seen as wholly undesirable, as tautological phenomena, to be managed or eradicated. Amongst Cassel nurses, there is a belief that the experience of these phenomena is meaningful and that they can be used to communicate important elements of social reality. If these communications can be registered and understood (Dartington, 1994), they can be contained (rather than controlled) and used to inform subsequent action. In this way, the sources of the original stress can become known, humanized, situated within a social context (Newton, 1995), and, therefore, experienced as less overwhelming and less persecutory.

Nurses are not regarded as having or behaving as if they have limitless resources and tolerance. Indeed, the reality of personal and professional limits and the possibility of saying 'No', challenge both the omnipotence of the professional carer and the desire for absolute dependency to be found in the regressed part of the patient.

Clinical and managerial supervision (Hinshelwood, 1979; Hawkins and Shohet, 1989) is considered to be crucial if psychosocial nurses are to develop an understanding and a capacity to manage themselves and others in relation to all of the above points. This has a multidisciplinary aspect in the practice of nurse–therapist supervision (Leach, 1987; Tischler, 1987).

Knowledge, skills and attitudes

An ability is developed to consider the psychodynamic/psychosocial significance and symbolic awareness of the postures, gestures, thinking, emotions and behaviour of individuals, in everyday life, at *individual* (Salzberger-Wittenberg, 1970; Pedder and Brown, 1991), *group* (Bion, 1961; Main, 1975; Turquet, 1985; Hinshelwood, 1987; Wright, 1989) and *organizational levels* (Colman and Bexton, 1974; Colman and Geller, 1985; DeBoard, 1978; Menzies-Lyth, 1988, 1989a,b; Armstrong, 1991; Obholzer and Roberts, 1994). This includes an ability to utilize these knowledge bases in understanding and working with personal and interpersonal communications in the different settings.

A psychodynamic and sociopsychological knowledge of human development (Winnicott, 1964, 1971; Erikson, 1977; Rayner, 1986), and an ability to use this knowledge, are needed to assess an individual's or a group's level of developmental functioning at any given time (short term or longer term) and to plan care and work accordingly.

An ability truly to observe, become aware of and listen to others' and to one's own thoughts, feelings and intuitions, and to use these in a spontaneous yet professional way, help to make therapeutic sense of reactive thoughts and feelings and to channel these into therapeutic responses. Nurses need to develop the ability to think with others when under pressure to act (be that internally or externally driven), to tolerate the uncertainty of not knowing and of appearing not to know, and to resist the pressure not to think, but merely act.

A knowledge of the history, influences (historical and contemporary) differing philosophies and views about therapeutic community approaches to care and treatment (Kennard, 1988, 1993; Manning, 1989). What is as important is a knowledge of the psychological components of management, of people, of oneself in a role, and of groups and organizations (Miller, 1993).

Conclusion

Aggleton and Chalmers (1987) advocate the need for a way of assessing and comparing nursing models. They suggest that the models differ in predictive power, have different implicit values, understand people and their problems from particular viewpoints, have different goals, deal with particular groups and differing degrees of holism. They also suggest that the models can be grouped (after Fawcett) into interactionist (based on symbolic interactionism), developmental and systemic types (although these differences are often relative).

The Cassel psychosocial model has certainly emerged out of a particular treatment setting, working with a particular group of patients, but that does not limit its applicability to that setting. It is developmental in that it strives towards achieving maturity, be that of an individual, a family, a group or a system. It is interactionist in that it seeks to understand complex personal, interpersonal, group and intergroup dynamics as meaningful communications, which may promote greater individual or collective understanding; it is systemic in terms of its objectives and methods.

Nursing theory is a framework to help nurses to think about what they do. Nursing models have made a contribution to that body of theory and will continue to do so, yet it is inconceivable that any model will become universal, nor is it probably desirable that this should be so. Even so, the validity and, perhaps more importantly, the applicability of a particular model can be judged in relation to increasingly accepted criteria. Fawcett's metaparadigm concepts of nursing (environment, health, person and nursing) have gained some agreement among nurses, as being of central concern to nursing (Walker, 1971; Flaskerud and Halloran, 1980).

The model of psychosocial nursing described in this chapter meets Fawcett's criteria, in that it consists of unifying statements encompassing all four concepts of the metaparadigm of nursing: nursing itself, the environment, the person, and the concept of health. It highlights, in complex ways, the interconnectedness of these four concepts, rather than relying on a focus on the relationship between a combination of pairs of the concepts (for example, health and the person, the person and the nurse, the nurse and health). It is important that it does not differentiate artificially the nurse from the other three concepts of person, health and environment. Instead, it situates the nurse centrally within and as part of this matrix, affected by it and affecting it. The patient and the nurse may have similar types of experience, this may all too often remain denied, projected or otherwise unused in traditional nursing systems. Indeed, it is the nurse's developed ability to use this experience reflexively in nursing work, which enables empathy with the patient.

Another pitfall of most models was identified and criticized by Jennings, et al. (1988). This concerns what they term an 'autonomy paradigm', which stresses an individualistic moral perspective, which establishes at its core the promotion of individual (person) autonomy and the protection of individual rights. This focuses on the relationship between person, health and nurse, but neglects the effects of, or the possibilities that exist within, the communal environment, the concept of interdependence and of the balancing of individual rights with collective responsibilities. In many treatment settings, attention is not paid to the features of the whole setting. Problems, ill health and difficulties are often located within the person (usually, discourses linked to an organic medical conceptual model (James, 1992)). Yet, if close attention is paid to the dynamic interrelatedness between the environment, the prevailing concept of health, the concept of the person (their family and immediate surroundings) and the concept of nurse (and nursing), this interrelatedness can be used as a therapeutic tool (and not merely seen as some random background to treatment), and new possibilities emerge.

Nursing in a therapeutic community is effective to the very extent that these four concepts can be interrelated and can be worked with consequently. The fact that the practitioners, as well as the recipients, of such nursing care generated the model, further validates its authority to say what psychosocial nursing is, and confirms its social relevance. The model has simply made explicit the embedded theory that has informed psychosocial nursing.

On reflection, what has been achieved in the development of this model is the arrangement of a set of philosophical claims about psychosocial nursing into a particular structure. These philosophical claims are a set of beliefs about what are the basic entities of psychosocial nursing at the hospital, how these entities are known and what values guide its practice. As Rew (1994: p. 23) suggests, they represent: 'not a single idea but the embodiment of collective and individual experiences, a dialectic between the human *being* and the human *doing*'.

However, the term 'model' suggests a rather fixed state of affairs and does not reflect the dynamic flux. Definitions of health and desirable qualities in patients are socially structured, culturally bound and change over time. A set of beliefs and values exist within the culture of nursing at the Cassel Hospital and these are taught through seminars and learnt through the daily engagement in nursing practice, but this is by no means a closed system of beliefs. They are challenged, affected and transformed by the prevailing cultural norms and by the beliefs patients, nurses and other staff bring to this culture. They are constantly being reinterpreted, reworked and revised. In making these beliefs and propositions explicit, there is a danger that they then might become the bench mark of psychosocial practice, to quote Main (1990: p. 64), 'mere beliefs, sets of never-to-be-questioned, always-to-be-believed rules, which now handicap further thought'.

Why, then, present these beliefs now? They are beliefs which the authors think and feel might usefully be applied and tried in other settings (Barber, 1988), perhaps particularly in other mental health care settings. In making explicit these beliefs about psychosocial nursing, it is hoped that three objectives have been achieved: first, a perspective for *practice*, by identifying the focus and goals of practice and delineating the values that guide both the practice and the psychosocial practitioner; secondly, a perspective for *research*, by identifying the phenomena central to psychosocial practice; and, thirdly, a perspective for *scholarship*, in that this will provide a point of reference for thinking, discussion and debate (Salsberry, 1994).

From a rhetorical point of view, these beliefs and ideas belong to a specific place and time. The authors believe that only through engaging with them emotionally and intellectually, through experimentation in practice, can they be truly known and an assessment made about their continued utility.

References

Aggleton, P. and Chalmers, H. (1987). Models of nursing, nursing practice and nurse education. *J. Adv. Nurs.* 12, 573–581.

Ahrenfeldt, R.H. (1958). *Psychiatry in the British Army in the Second World War*. Routledge and Kegan Paul.

Armstrong, D. (1991). *The Institution in the Mind: Reflections on the Relation of Psychoanalysis to Work with Institutions* (and postscript). Grubb Institute.

Barber, P. (1988). Learning to grow: the necessity for educational processing in therapeutic community practice. *Int. J. Ther. Communities*, 9(2), 101–108.

Barnes, E. ed. (1968). *Psychosocial Nursing: Studies from the Cassel Hospital*. Tavistock Publications.

Benner, P. (1984). *From Novice to Expert: Excellence and Power in Clinical Nursing Practice*. Addison-Wesley.

Bion, W. (1961). *Experiences in Groups*. Tavistock Publications.

Bion, W. (1970). *Attention and Interpretation*. Tavistock Publications.

Bridger, H. (1985). Northfield revisited. In *Bion and Group Psychotherapy* (M. Pines, ed.) pp. 87–107, Routledge and Kegan Paul.

Casey, P.R. and Tyrer, P.J. (1986). Personality, functioning and symptomatology. *Journal of Psychiatric Research*, 20, 363–374.

Chapman, G.E. (1984). A therapeutic community, psychosocial nursing and the nursing process. *Int. J. Ther. Communities*, 5(2), 68–76.

Chapman, G.E. (1988a). Reporting therapeutic discourse in a therapeutic community. *J. Adv. Nurs. Stud.*, 13, 255–264.

Chapman, G.E. (1988b). Text, talk and discourse in a therapeutic community. *Int. J. Ther. Communities*, 9(2): 75–87.

Chiesa, M., Iacoponi, E. and Morris, M. (1996). Changes in health service utilisation by patients with severe personality disorders before and after inpatient psychosocial treatment. *Br. J. Psychother.*, 12, 501–512.

Clarke, L. (1988). Ideology, tradition and choice: questions psychiatric nurses ask themselves. *Senior Nurse*, 8: 11–13.

Colman, A.D. and Bexton, W.H. (1974). *Group Relations Reader 1*. GREX.

Colman, A.D. and Geller, M.H. (1985). *Group Relations Reader 2*. (A.K. Rice Institute Series.) A.K. Rice Institute.

Conran, M. (1991). Running on the spot, or can nursing really change? Response to Julia Fabricius. *Psychoanal. Psychother.*, 5, 109–114.

Dartington, A. (1994). Where angels fear to tread. In *The Unconscious at Work* (A. Obholzer and V. Roberts, eds) pp. 101–109, Routledge.

DeBoard, R. (1978). *The Psychoanalysis of Organizations*. Tavistock Publications.

de Lambert, L. (1982). The Role of a nurse in a psychotherapeutic institution. In *Psychotherapie in der Klinik* (H. Hilpert, F. Schwartz and F. Beese, eds) pp. 114–122, Springer-Verlag.

Denford, J. and Griffiths, P. (1993). 'Transferences to the institution' and their effect on inpatient treatment at the Cassel Hospital. *Ther. Communities*, 14, 237–248.

Dolan, B. Evans, C. and Wilson, J. (1992). Therapeutic community treatment for personality disordered adults: changes in neurotic symptomatology on follow up. *Inter. J. Soc. Psychiatry*, 38, 242–250.

Downie, R. (1990). Ready, steady, stop? *Soc. Work Today*, 12 July, 9.

Draper, J. (1992). The impact of nursing models. *Senior Nurse*, 12(3), 38–39.

Erikson, E. (1977). *Childhood and Society*. Paladin Books.

Fabricius, J. (1991). Running on the spot, or can nursing really change? *Psychoanal. Psychother.*, 5, 97–108.

Fawcett, J. (1984). *Analysis and Evaluation of Conceptual Models of Nursing*. Davis.

Flaskerud, J.H. and Halloran, E.J. (1980). Areas of agreement in nursing. *Adv. Nurs. Sci.*, 3(1), 1–7.

Flynn C. (1993). The patients' pantry: the nature of the nursing task. *Ther. Communities*, 14, 227–236.

Foucault, M. (1965). *Madness and Civilization: A History of Insanity in the Age of Reason*. Tavistock.

Foucault, M. (1973). *The Birth of the Clinic: An Archaeology of Medical Perception*. Tavistock.

Foucault, M. (1987). *Mental Illness and Psychology*. California Press.

Freud, S. (1961). Civilization and its discontents. In *The Complete works of Sigmund Freud*, vol. 21 (J. Strachey, ed.) pp. 64–145, Hogarth Press.

Gabbard, G.O. (1992). The therapeutic relationship in psychiatric hospital treatment. *Bull. Menninger Clin.*, 56(1), 4–9.

General Nursing Council for England and Wales. (1982). *Training Syllabus Register of Nurses, Mental Nursing*. London.

Goldie, L. (1991). Ethical dilemmas for nurses and their emotional implications. *Psychoanal. Psychother.*, 5, 125–138.

Greenwood, J. (1984) Nursing research: a position paper. *J. Adv. Nurs.*, 9, 77–82.

Griffiths, P. and Pringle, P. eds (1997). *Psychosocial Practice in a Residential Setting*. Karmac Books, London.

Habermas, J. and McCarthy, T. (1976). *Communication and the Evolution of Society*. Beacon.

Hale, R. and Campbell, D. (1991). Suicidal acts. In *A Textbook of Psychotherapy in Psychiatric Practice* (J. Holmes, ed.) pp. 287–306, Churchill Livingstone.

Haque, G. (1973). Psychosocial nursing in the community. *Nurs. Times*, (13 Jan).

Hawkins, P. and Shohet, R. (1989). *Supervision in the Helping Professions*. Open University Press.

Hinshelwood, R.D. (1979). Supervision as an exchange system. In *Therapeutic Communities: Reflections and Progress* (R.D. Hinshelwood and N. Manning, eds.) Section G: Research, pp. 208–219, Routledge and Kegan Paul.

Hinshelwood, R.D. (1987). *What Happens in Groups: Psychoanalysis, the Individual and the Community*. Free Association Books.

Hinshelwood, R. D. and Griffiths, P. (1997). Actions speak louder than words. In *Psychosocial Practice in a Residential Setting* (P. Griffiths and P. Pringle, eds.). Karnac Books, London.

Hinshelwood, R.D. and Manning, N. (1979). *Therapeutic Communities – Reflections and Progress*. Routledge and Kegan Paul.

Hiraki, A. (1992). Tradition, rationality and power in introductory nursing textbooks: a critical hermeneutics study. *Adv. Nurs. Sci.*, 14(3), 1–12.

Holter, M.I. and Schwartz-Barcot, D. (1993). Action research: what is it? How has it been used and how can it be used in nursing? *J. Adv. Nurs.*, 18, 298–304.

Hughes, P.M. and Halek, C. (1991). Training nurses in psychotherapeutic skills. *Psychoanal. Psychother.*, 5, 115–123.

Irwin, F. (1995). The therapeutic ingredients in baking a cake. *Ther. Communities*, 16, 263–268.

Jackson, M. and Cawley, R. (1992). Psychodynamics and psychotherapy on an acute psychiatric ward. *Br. J. Psychiatry*, 160, 41–50.

Jackson, M. and Willaims, P. (1994). *Unimaginable Storms: a Search for Meaning in Psychosis*. Karnac Books.

James, N. (1992). Care = organisation + physical labour + emotional labour. *Sociol. Health Illness*. 14(4), 488–509.

38 Models and frameworks

James, O. (1987). The role of the nurse/therapist relationship in the therapeutic community. In *The Family as In-patient* (R. Kennedy, A. Heymann and L. Tischler, eds.) pp. 78–94, Free Association Books.

James, O. and Wilson, A. (1987). A sexually charged clinical problem: social, structural and classical psychoanalytic approaches. In *The Family as In-patient* (R. Kennedy, A. Heymann and L. Tischler, eds.) pp. 315–328, Free Association Books.

Jaques, E. (1960). Disturbances in the capacity to work. *Int. J. Psychoanal.* **XLI**, parts 4–5, 357–367.

Jennings, B., Callahan, D. and Caplan, A. (1988). Ethical challenge of chronic illness. *Hastings Center Report*, **18**(1) (special suppl.), 1–16. Cited in Salsberry, P.L. (1984). A philosophy of nursing: what is it? what it is not? In *Developing a Philosophy of Nursing* (J.F. Kikuchi and H. Simmons, eds.), Sage.

Kennard, D. (1988). The therapeutic community. In *Group Therapy in Britain* (A. Aveline and W. Dryden, eds.) pp. 153–184, Open University Press.

Kennard, D. (1993). The future revisited: new frontiers for the therapeutic community concept. *Ther. Communities*, **15**, 107–113.

Kennedy, R. (1987a). Introduction. In *The family as In-patient* (R. Kennedy, A. Heymans and L. Tischler, eds.) pp. 1–24, Free Association Books.

Kennedy, R. (1987b). Work of the day. In *The Family as In-patient* (R. Kennedy, A. Heymans, and L. Tischler, eds.) pp. 27–48, Free Association Books.

Kennedy, R., Heymans, A. and Tischler, L. (1987). *The Family as In-patient*. Free Association Books.

Kenny, T. (1993). Nursing models fail in practice. *Br. J. Nurs.*, **2**(2), 133–136.

Klein, M. (1975). *The Writings of Melanie Klein. Vol. 1: Love, Guilt and Reparation*, pp. 128–138, Hogarth.

Lacey, D.G. (1993). Discovering theory from psychiatric nursing practice. *Br. J. Nurs.*, **2**, 763–766.

Leach, G. (1987). Nurse/therapist supervision as an impetus to change. In *The Family as In-patient* (R. Kennedy, A. Heymans and L. Tischler, eds.) pp. 160–166, Free Association Books.

Lewis, G. and Appleby, S. (1988). Personality disorders: the patients psychiatrists dislike. *Br. J. Psychiatry*, **153**, 44–49.

Lundh, U. Soder, M. and Waemess, K. (1988). Nursing theories: a critical view. *Image*, **20**, 222–224.

McCaffrey, G. (1994). An account of outreach nursing at the Cassel. *Ther. Communities*, **15**(3), 173–181.

Macklin, D. (1979). Trouble stirring in the kitchen. *Nurs. Times*, (24 May).

Main, T.F. (1946). The hospital as a therapeutic institution. *Bull. Menninger Clin.*, **10**(3), 66–70.

Main, T. (1957). The ailment. *Br. J. Med. Psychol.*, **30**, 129–145.

Main, T.F. (1967). Knowledge, learning and freedom from thought. *Aust. N. Z. J. Psychiatry*, **1**(2), 64–71.

Main, T. (1975). Some dynamics of large groups. In *The Large Group* (L. Kreeger, ed.) pp. 57–86, Constable.

Main, T.F. (1983). The concept of a therapeutic community: variations and vicissitudes. In *The Evolution of Group Analysis* (M. Pines, ed.) pp. 197–217,

Routledge and Kegan Paul.

Main, T.F. (1989). The concept of a therapeutic community. In *The Ailment and Other Psychoanalytic Essays* (Main, T.F.: J. Johns, ed.) pp. 123–141, Free Association Books.

Main, T.F. (1990). Knowledge, learning and freedom from thought. *Psychoanal. Psychother.*, 5, 59–78.

Manning, N. (1979). The politics of survival: the role of research in the therapeutic community. In *Therapeutic Communities: Reflections and Progress* (R. D. Hinshelwood and N. Manning, eds.) pp. 287–296, Routledge and Kegan Paul.

Manning, N. (1989). The origins of the therapeutic community. In *The Therapeutic Community Movement: Charisma and Routinization* (N. Manning, ed.) pp. 1–28, Routledge.

Manthey, M. (1980). *The Practice of Primary Nursing*. Blackwell Scientific.

Meinrath, M.R. and Roberts, J. (1982). On being a good enough staff member. *Int. J. Ther. Communities*, 3(1), 7–14.

Menzies, I.E.P. (1960). A case study in the functioning of a social system as a defence against anxiety. *Hum. Relations*, 13, 95–121. (Reprinted as Tavistock Pamphlet 3, 1970.)

Menzies-Lyth, I.E.P. (1988). *Containing Anxiety in Institutions. (Selected Essays, vol. 1)*. Free Association Books.

Menzies-Lyth, I.E.P. ed. (1989a). *The Dynamics of the Social*. Free Association Books.

Menzies-Lyth, I. (1989b). A personal review of group experiences. Bion's contribution to thinking about groups. In *The Dynamics of the Social* (I. Menzies-Lyth, ed.) pp. 19–25, Free Association Books.

Miller, E. (1993). Innovation in a psychiatric hospital. In *From Dependency to Autonomy – Studies in Organisations and Change* (E. Miller, ed.) pp. 217–237, Free Association Books.

Morrice, J.K.W. (1979). Basic concepts: a critical review. In *Therapeutic Communities – Reflections and Progress* (R. Hinshelwood and N. Manning, eds.) pp. 49–58, Routledge and Kegan Paul.

Newton, T. (1995). *'Managing' Stress, emotion and power at work*. Sage.

Obholzer, A. and Roberts, V. (1994). *The Unconscious at Work*. Routledge.

Oldman, J. (1995). Outcomes research: results update. *The Cassel Newsletter*, 2(Oct), 2–3.

Orem, D. (1980). *Nursing Concepts in Practice*, second edition. McGraw Hill.

Pearson, A. and Vaughan, B. (1986). *Nursing Models for Practice*. Heinemann.

Pedder, J. and Brown, D. (1991). *Introduction to Psychotherapy: an Outline of Psychodynamic Principles and Practice*. Routledge.

Peplau, H.E. (1952). *Interpersonal Relations in Nursing*. Putnam.

Peplau, H.E. (1994). Psychiatric mental health nursing. *J. Psychiatr. Ment. Health Nurs.*, 1, 3–7.

Ploye, P. (1977). On some difficulties of in-patient psychoanalytically orientated therapy. *Psychiatry*, 40, 133–145.

Rapoport, R.N. (1960). *The Community as Doctor: New Perspectives on a Therapeutic Community*. Tavistock Publications.

Rayner, E. (1986). *Human Development*. Allen and Unwin.

Reason, P. ed. (1988). *Human Inquiry in Action: Developments in New Paradigm Research*. Sage.

Rew, L. (1994). Commentary. In *Developing a Philosophy of Nursing*. (J.F. Kikuchi and H. Simmons, eds.) pp. 20–24, Sage.

Roberts, V. (1994). The self assigned impossible task. In *The Unconscious at Work* (A. Obholzer and V. Roberts, eds.) pp. 110–118, Routledge.

Robinson, S. (1994). Life after death. *Ther. Communities*, 15, 77–86.

Rose, N. (1985). *The Psychological Complex*. Routledge and Kegan Paul.

Rose, N. (1989). *Governing the Soul*. Routledge.

Ross, T.A. (1923). *The Common Neurosis*. Edward Arnold.

Ross, T.A. (1932). *An Introduction to Analytical Psychotherapy*. Edward Arnold.

Ross, T.A. (1936). *An Enquiry into the Prognosis of Neurosis*. Cambridge University Press.

Rosser, R.M, Birch, S. and Bond, H. (1987). Five year follow-up of patients treated with in-patient psychotherapy at the Cassel Hospital. *J. R. Soc. Med.*, 80, 549–555.

Salsberry, P.L. (1994). A philosophy of nursing: What is it? What it is not? In *Developing a Philosophy of Nursing* (J.F. Kikuchi and H. Simmons, eds.) pp. 11–19, Sage.

Salzberger-Wittenberg, I. (1970). *Psychoanalytic Insights and Relationships*. Routledge.

Schroder, P.J. (1985). Recognising transference and countertransference *J. Psychosoc. Nurs.*, 23(2), 21–25.

Sheehan, J. (1996). Managed change or management speak. *Nurs. Times*, 92(13), 42–44.

Siegler, M. and Osmond, H. (1976). *Models of Madness, Models of Medicine*. Macmillan.

Stanton, A. and Schwartz, M. (1954). *The Mental Hospital*. Basic Books.

Tischler, L. (1987). Nurse therapist supervision. In *The Family as In-patient* (R. Kennedy, A. Heymans and L. Tischler, eds.) pp. 95–107, Free Association Books.

Tonnesman, M. (1979). Containing stress in professional work: the human encounter in the caring professions. *Social Work Service Magazine* (DHSS) 21, 34–41.

Towell, D. and Harries, C. (1979). *Innovation in Patient Care: An Action Research Study of Change in a Psychiatric Hospital*. Croom Helm.

Trent, D.R. (1992). Breaking the single continuum. In *Promotion of Mental Health*, vol. 1 (D.R. Trent, ed.) pp. 117–126, Avebury.

Turquet, P.M. (1985). Leadership: the individual and the group. In *Group Relations Reader 2* (A.D. Colman and M.H. Geller, eds.) pp. 71–87, A.K. Rice Institute.

Tyrer, P. ed. (1988). *Personality Disorders: Diagnosis, Management and Cause*. Wright.

Tyrer, P.J., Casey, P.R. and Ferguson, B. (1993). Personality disorder in perspective. In *Personality Disorder Reviewed* (P.J. Tyrer and G. Stein, eds.) pp. 1–16, Gaskell, Royal College of Psychiatrists.

van der Linden, P. (1988). How does the large group change the individual? *Int. J. Ther. Communities*, 9(1), 31–39.

Walker, L.O. (1971). Toward a clearer understanding of the concept of nursing theory. *Nurs. Res.*, **20**, 428–435.

Weddell, D. (1955). Psychology as applied to nursing. (A series of notes for tutors and others concerned in the training of student nurses.) *Nurs. Times*, Sep 1954 – Mar 1955.

Weddell, D. (1968). Change of approach. In *Psychosocial Nursing: Studies from the Cassel Hospital* (E. Barnes, ed.) pp. 61–72, Tavistock Publications.

Winnicott, W. (1964). *The Child, the Family and the Outside World*, Penguin.

Winnicott, W. (1965). The theory of parent infant relationship. The development of the capacity to be alone. From dependence towards independence in the development of the individual. The mentally ill in your caseload. Chapters in *The Maturational Processes and the Facilitating Environment*, Hogarth Press.

Winnicott, W. (1971). *Playing and Reality*. Tavistock Publications.

Winship, G. (1995). Nursing and psychoanalysis – uneasy alliances. *Psychoanal. Psychother.* **9**, 289–299.

Wright, H. (1989). *Group work: Perspectives and Practice*. Scutari.

Wright, H. (1991). The patient, the nurse, his life and her mother: psychodynamic influences in nurse education and practice. *Psychoanal. Psychother.*, **5**, 139–149.

Chapter 2

Subjective experience and social enquiry

Jacqueline Ord

This chapter outlines an approach to social enquiry which values subjective experience. I suggest that such an approach has much to offer nurses, and to others who work with suffering people. These ideas can also be useful for managers in settings that need to take account of people's emotional distress. All organizations need to do this to some extent, but the human services (especially those that deal with people in emotional crises) need to pay serious attention to the implications of this distress in the way they operate (Obholzer, 1994). I suggest that nurses and managers, as well as researchers, might understand and use methods of enquiry based on direct observation, that they should attend to information gained through personal experience, and that they should understand the philosophical basis that justifies such an approach.

Some examples from my own experience will be used. As a nurse at the Cassel Hospital, I learnt how to use my emotional reactions to patients to develop my clinical practice, and later, as a social scientist, I applied this learning to research issues of culture and communication in a large urban health district. The focus for the research was the installation of a district-wide computer network. The expensive new system failed to deliver, due to organizational, rather than technical, problems: a classic case of what not to do when introducing change, and a classic case of the users not being consulted.

Such failures can be useful. They make visible the processes by which organizations, like individuals, seem to defend themselves against painful feelings by denying their importance. Learning through shared reflection becomes impossible, relationships are fragmented and mistrustful, the quest for efficiency justifies greed and leads to waste, and the administration undermines, rather than supports, people working at the clinical interface.

Whether we work at a clinical or an institutional level, as practitioners or researchers (hopefully both), the capacity to acknowledge, discuss and learn from our emotional reactions is vital if we are to create environments in which troubled people, and those who care for them, can feel sufficiently held and supported.

Logic versus emotion: control at all costs?

The UK National Health Service (NHS) has been frequently reorganized for purposes of management control. These reorganizations have left nurses with little say over how resources should be used; successive reorganizations put nurses under increasing pressure, while increasing resources were devoted to managerial functions (Osborne, 1993). Obholzer (1994: p. 173) suggests that such constant reorganization in NHS institutions can be seen as a way of defending against the fact that they exist to help people to cope with desperately painful situations: 'The new style of management is to give managers power and to eliminate consultation as "inefficient" . . . fragmenting and splitting up systems instead of promoting collaboration.' He argues that this denial, paradoxically, leads to more and more inefficiency.

Nurse education, since Project 2000 (United Kingdom Central Council for Nursing Midwifery and Health Visiting, 1986), is aimed at producing nurses who are 'knowledgeable doers'. Fabricius (1991) says:

> In the emphasis on *knowing* and *doing*, a third mode of function, namely *being*, seems to have been entirely neglected. Because I would submit that the nurses' ability to *be*, with and for the patient, is the most important way in which he needs her to be psychotherapeutic.

By psychotherapeutic, Fabricius means the capacity of the nurse to help patients to bear feelings of overwhelming anxiety and distress, by acting as a 'container' for such feelings (to use an idea from Winnicott, 1965). She points out, however, that this function is often impossible for the nurse to carry out unless the nurse, too, feels held or contained within an appropriate institutional context. Rather than supporting this vital nursing function, however, health care institutions have reduced their support while increasing their demands on nurses. Fabricius describes:

> . . . the very fast through-put of patients compared with a few years ago: the awful physical environment and lack of resources which many nurses are working in and with: the general poor morale and feeling among nurses that they are not valued: the lack of really senior and experienced nurses still working in the wards: and the changed management structures in hospitals.'

Reflexivity, philosophy and social research

The opposition between logic and emotion within the NHS is supported by the wider social and economic context. At the heart of Western industrial culture lies a deep split between thought and feeling. This duality lies also at the heart of a long-standing academic debate between two opposing perspectives: positivism and subjectivism. Positivists are concerned with objectivity, see the world as separate from themselves, and argue that subjective experience is unreliable. Subjectivists, on the other hand, argue that the observer is a key element in the scientific process, and that the researcher's subjective experience is a central focus of enquiry.

The validity of emotional responses in understanding other people is taken for granted in psychoanalytical theory, where emotion is seen as a fundamental way of knowing and relating. Such understanding has not, however, been esteemed as having high scientific status in the Western world (Smail, 1984). Traditionally, the objective stance has been the hallmark of scientific research. The data are 'out there' and the researcher's job is to observe and analyse these data in an attempt to prove or disprove theoretical hypotheses. In many cases, however, where theoretical frameworks need to be constructed, it is argued that researchers need to build a 'grounded theory' based on direct observation of the social world (Glaser and Strauss, 1978).

Research that uses this kind of direct observation is usually referred to as ethnography, or participant observation. Although a variety of techniques can be used, from interviews to acting a role, a central requirement is that the researcher creates and maintains face-to-face relationships with people in the natural context of their daily lives.

The philosophical approach which justifies ethnographic research is a branch of existentialism known as phenomenology (literally, the study of 'phenomena'). Phenomenology provides a solution to a philosophical argument which has raged in Western cultures for thousands of years

(Magee, 1987: p. 254): whether or not objects of our consciousness have a separate existence from us, independent of our experience of them. The phenomenological stance resolves this argument by pointing out that, whatever existential status objects may or may not have, there can be no doubt that they exist as objects of consciousness for us, and we can therefore investigate them on this basis without having to concern ourselves with questions about their independent existence. What is more, we have direct and immediate access to the objects of our consciousness, and therefore are in the best possible position to find out about them. Phenomenology sees an individual's subjective experience as the prime focus for studying the social world. This perspective allows direct access to the interplay between internal and external experience, and has as its goal the systematic understanding of the way we create meaning between one another. These ideas have influenced work in the sociology of knowledge, such as Berger and Luckman's (1979) argument that what we take for granted as 'reality' is in fact socially constructed through our day-to-day interactions. These interactions become so familiar that they are hardly noticed, until a stranger asks questions that others would never think to ask. In ethnography, the researcher's role is like that of a stranger learning how to become a part of a newly-met culture. In the process, the researcher aims to make explicit those taken-for-granted ways of interacting that normally go unnoticed, but which enable people to create and sustain a shared reality. Researchers, then, have no choice but to become part of the social system they are studying, and are required to examine their subjective experience as a way of understanding that social system. This self-examination is known by ethnographers as 'reflexivity' (Whyte, 1943; Sanday, 1979; Hammersley and Atkinson, 1995). Hammersley and Atkinson refer to the researcher as:

> The research instrument *par excellence* . . . This is not a matter of methodological commitment, it is an existential fact. There is no way in which we can escape the social world in order to study it; nor fortunately, is that necessary . . . How people respond to the presence of the researcher may be as informative as how they react to other situations (pp. 14–15).

The capacity for reflection on experience – which I too shall call 'reflexivity' – is central to social research methods which rely on direct observation of people in their natural environments. These methods, I suggest, have great value in understanding the links between social systems and individual behaviour.

Over the last two decades of the twentieth century, the emotional work of nurses has been a topic of particular interest to a growing number of researchers who are aiming to make explicit the knowledge and understanding that nurses use in their everyday practice (Lawler, 1991; Smith, 1992; Savage, 1995). They use methods of ethnography, or participant observation, since their concern is to understand the way people make sense of their natural environment, whether it be at home, at work, or in a clinical setting. The nurse's and the ethnographer's tasks are similar in that both are crucially about face-to-face interaction and direct observation, and both require the capacity to acknowledge and reflect on subjective data.

The question for care workers, managers and researchers alike, is how to maintain a reflexive stance which allows us constantly to examine our taken-for-granted assumptions. This requires ongoing support and skills development, which are best sustained by an institutional 'culture of enquiry', in which feelings and thoughts, rather than being seen as opposites, can inform one another: a culture which 'both requires and sanctions . . . enquiry into personal and interpersonal and intersystem . . . relations as these are expressed and arranged socially' (Main, 1989: p. 141).

Learning from experience: the use of reflexivity in psychosocial nursing

Within the culture of enquiry at the Cassel Hospital, the course in psychosocial nursing provides an excellent grounding in reflexivity and participant observation. Nurses, on a daily basis, try to understand the behaviour of people, principally patients, but also colleagues, and, of course, themselves. It is taken for granted in psychosocial nursing that the best way to understand someone is to work alongside him or her in a common task. Thus, it is through sharing the apparently mundane jobs of cleaning the common room, or shopping for children's teas, that nurses learn about patients' patterns of relating. In order to sustain their capacity to learn, and to work sensitively with very challenging patients, Weddell (1968) recognized that nurses need frequent, formalized, opportunities to reflect on their work, and to explore strainful situations with colleagues. Psychosocial nursing with patients at the Cassel Hospital is, therefore, interspersed with a systematic programme of nurse meetings, seminars and interdisciplinary team meetings.

The following examples, taken from my own experience at the Cassel Hospital, illustrate how psychosocial nurse training develops one's abilities to observe others, to understand one's own reactions, and to use these insights in tolerating and working with people in distress.

I often found that mealtimes in the family dining room were difficult to tolerate. Mothers were often angry with their children, and my sympathies would be with the little ones who, I felt, were being heavily punished for trivial reasons. I found it extremely difficult to know how to interact with mothers who seemed so unreasonable, and felt very critical of their mothering. However, in tutorials on human psychological development, and through discussions with colleagues, I came to appreciate that the sense of despair I felt at mealtimes was a reflection of the despair felt by the mothers. I became aware of how important it was not to side with the children, but to find ways of supporting the mothers, who had usually experienced inadequate nurturing in their own childhood. This helped me to tolerate the mothers' behaviour and to find ways of supporting them, rather than being critical.

The next example shows in more detail how reflection with colleagues can help nurses to understand their emotional responses to patients. I was on night duty when a young woman, Christine, cut her wrists. The cuts were deep and I called in the duty doctor, who advised me to take her to the casualty department of the local hospital for suturing. Christine said she wanted to go to her room and change before we went, but I was anxious that she would harm herself further, if not kill herself. It was only after an argument with her, that I relented and allowed her the privacy of her room in which to change her clothes. Later, in a nursing seminar, I talked about this very distressing incident and my fear that Christine would kill herself. The seminar leader suggested that my fear was, in fact, my own projected wish that she would do so. I felt a shock of recognition and, with the support of my colleagues, I became aware of the murderous feelings that underlay my anxiety. When, later, another patient cut herself, I felt I handled the situation much better. I was able to be open with her about my angry feelings, and was then able to feel and show sympathy for the distress which lay behind her hurting herself.

An example of ethnographic research in a district health authority

At the Cassel Hospital, the culture of enquiry facilitates openness and mutual support. This provides an institutional framework which has the capacity to hold and contain the potentially overwhelming anxieties of clients and of staff. This is not the case, unfortunately, in many areas of the NHS. In this section, I describe some ethnographic research I carried out in a large health district, Greyborough, which was installing a Medilink system, a networked computer system with over 300 terminals situated at a variety of clinical and administrative sites. (Pseudonyms are used to preserve anonymity.) The aim of the research was to develop grounded theories about the organizational, social and cultural issues involved in installing this kind of large computer network in a health district.

My previous nursing background helped me to gain access to the project site and, in my role as researcher, I attended meetings between Magnatel (the computer company), Greyborough administrators, and representatives from the regional health authority and the Department of Health. The region and the department between them had invested many thousands of pounds in the project, and were keen to evaluate its potential benefits for other health districts. I was offered a job as system evaluator, and, after consideration, I took it on a part-time basis. This would allow me to work alongside the project team, which I knew from my Cassel experience would give me access to richer data than I would obtain from mere observation.

Magnatel, with the help of a retired medical consultant, had sold the Medilink system to Greyborough District on the grounds that it would generate statistical information which could be used by managers for purposes of financial control. There was pressure from the Government at that time that the NHS should begin to cost its services. It was claimed, moreover, that the district's serious communications problems (these were never defined) would be alleviated by the ability of staff to communicate via computer terminals.

In taking on a formal role as a member of the project evaluation team, I became subject to the kinds of pressure which members of the team were facing. On one hand, there was pressure from senior managers within Greyborough and Magnatel to promote the project as successful and beneficial. On the other, direct observation of staff attempting to use the system revealed their cynicism and frustration at having their own communication systems disrupted. The clinical staff had not been adequately consulted at the design stage. The district nurses, in particular, found that the computer system undermined their carefully worked out methods of paper-based communication. It was only when they were on site that Magnatel staff comprehended the problems that this lack of consultation was to create. Despite their feelings of dismay and frustration at the 'negativity' of their potential users, they put on brave faces at formal meetings and insisted that they were 'ahead of the game'. The relationships within and between the teams concerned with the system were very fragmented and unstable. The evaluation team, for example, had a new chairperson and new members at almost every meeting. There was a difference of opinion between the project team, who were responsible for installing the system, and the evaluation team, who were responsible for evaluating its costs and benefits. The evaluation team tried to get the installation team to confront the fact that the project had failed, but the installation team denied there was anything wrong. They insisted that the installation was a success and attacked the evaluation team for being overcritical. In the formal meetings where these issues were discussed, there was no place for exploring feelings and impressions; plans, figures and targets were the order of the day. Feelings were perceived as obstacles to progress, rather than as important data to be explored. Behind the scenes, though, many of the people involved expressed frustration, dismay and anxiety.

The Medilink system was systematically sabotaged by hospital staff who, after some weeks of playing with sending jokey messages to each other, virtually gave up using it. The system was eventually dismantled, but not until after many hundreds of thousands of pounds had been wasted on the equipment, not to mention hundreds of hours of staff time spent in project meetings (Ord, 1989, 1996).

Discussion

The Medilink case illustrates how resources can be wasted in attempts to increase managerial control of finances. When nurses are excluded from management decisions, there is a danger that managers will waste resources that nurses need to provide adequate care. Nurses can best challenge such decisions if they have an institution-wide perspective on the way that resources are allocated, and the confidence to argue their case.

Nursing has traditionally been women's work, and women's work has traditionally been undervalued, ignored or, at best, taken for granted. It has also been taken for granted that women's role is to be concerned with emotional life and emotional needs, while men are concerned with facts, figures and logic (James, 1989, 1992). This split reflects the duality between logic and emotion which is a central feature of Western industrial culture. Within this culture generally, and certainly within the decision-making processes of the NHS, feelings (feminine, soft, intangible, messy, based in oral culture) are devalued in favour of rational thought (masculine, hard-nosed, factual, predictable, based in literacy).

As a researcher, the subjective experience of participating in the Medilink project was deeply disturbing. It was difficult to maintain a sense of personal integrity within the very split and fragmented relationships surrounding the new system. This subjective experience provides valuable data about what underlies the failure of many computer systems, within the NHS and elsewhere. New computer systems, like strangers, can reveal taken-for-granted ways of social interaction. What seemed taken-for-granted at Greyborough was the denial of human feelings. Beneath the facade of rationality, the managers' uncertainties, political manipulations, and fragmented relationships went unchallenged. Nurses gave up attending project meetings where their views and feelings were ignored, as were any views that challenged the viability of the system. The result was that over half a million pounds was wasted on computer equipment, which was either not used or was actively sabotaged by district staff. This was at a time when nurses were unable to obtain basic supplies such as clean linen, and when the state of the hospital kitchen caused a national scandal.

The Medilink case is by no means an isolated incident. Most notoriously, in the late 1980s, Wessex Regional Health Authority was severely criticized for its failed £43 million information technology strategy, where £20 million was wasted on their information systems plan.

One rationale for initiating the Medilink project was that it would provide an opportunity to learn from experience. I have used examples from my nursing at the Cassel Hospital to show how learning from experience, or reflexivity, as with other skills, needs to be developed and supported within an appropriate institutional culture. The culture of Greyborough Health District, however, provided little opportunity for open reflection and debate; it was quite the opposite. This suggests that nurses and researchers might need to look beyond the clinical arena, towards institutional factors that support or undermine their work. I would argue that, at an institutional level, the appropriate culture for the best use of resources is the same culture of enquiry that encourages reflexivity and open debate on clinical issues, a culture which supports nurses in their task of emotional holding for people in distress.

Ethnographic research can play a valuable role in developing such a culture of enquiry, in which difficult feelings can be acknowledged and contained: first by demonstrating the need for it through case studies such as Medilink; secondly, by arguing for philosophies and methods of enquiry that acknowledge the value of reflexivity and subjective experience; and, thirdly, by making explicit the value of nurses' subjective knowledge.

References

Berger, P. and Luckman, T. (1979). *The Social Construction of Reality. A Treatise in the Sociology of Knowledge.* Peregrine Books.

Fabricius, J. (1991). Running on the spot, or can nursing really change? *Psychoanal. Psychother.*, 5, 97–108.

Glaser, B. and Strauss, A. (1978). *The Discovery of Grounded Theory.* Weidenfeld and Nicolson.

Hammersley, M. and Atkinson, P. (1995). *Ethnography Principles in Practice.* Tavistock Publications.

James, N. (1989). Emotional labour, skills and work in the regulation of feelings. *Sociol. Rev.*, 37(1), 15–42.

James, N. (1992). Care = organisation + physical labour + emotional labour. *Sociol. Health Illness*, 14, 488–509.

Lawler, J. (1991). *Behind the Screens – Nursing, Somology and the Problem of the Body.* Churchill Livingstone.

Magee, B. (1987). *The Great Philosophers: An Introduction to Western Philosophy.* BBC Publications.

Main, T.F. (1989). The concept of a therapeutic community. In *The Ailment and Other Psychoanalytic Essays* (T.F. Main and J. Jones, eds.) p. 141, Free Association Books.

Obholzer, A. (1994) Managing social anxieties in public sector organizations. In *The Unconscious at Work: Individual and Organizational Stress in the Human Services* (A. Obholzer and V.Z. Roberts, eds.) p. 173, Routledge.

Ord, J. (1989). Who's joking? The information system at play. *Interact. Comput.*, 1, 118–128.

Osbourne, P. (1993). 5000 nurses go as managers are trebled. *London Evening Standard.*

Sanday, P.R. (1979). The ethnographic paradigms. *Admin. Sci. Q.*, 24, 527–538.

Savage, J. (1995). *Nursing Intimacy: an Ethnographic Approach to Nurse–Patient Interaction.* Scutari.

Smail, D. (1984). *Illusion and Reality: The Meaning of Anxiety.* Dent.

Smith, P. (1992). *The emotional labour of nursing. How nurses care.* Macmillan.

United Kingdom Central Council for Nursing Midwifery and Health Visiting. (1986). *Project 2000: A New Preparation for Practice.* UKCC.

Weddell, D. (1968). Change as a learning situation. In *Psychosocial Nursing: Studies from the Cassel Hospital* (E. Barnes, ed.) pp. 299–303, Tavistock Publications.

Whyte, W.F. (1943). *Street Corner Society*. University of Chicago Press.

Winnicott, D.W., ed. (1965). The maturational process and the facilitating environment. In *The Theory of the Parent–infant Relationship*. Hogarth.

Chapter 3

Implementing change: lessons learnt from the Cassel Hospital/Austen Riggs Center exchange programme

Mimi Francis

This chapter describes some lessons learned in the process of trying to change a nursing care system. The events occurred a number of years ago, but the lessons endure. My hope in recounting them here is to give some direction to another nurse somewhere who is trying to put into practice his or her vision of how things might be. The model used here is that of psychosocial nursing as developed and practised at the Cassel Hospital.

In the early 1970s I had the opportunity to undertake the Cassel Hospital course in psychological and family-centred nursing. In 1975 I began work at the Austen Riggs Center in Western Massachusetts, USA, with the task of developing a nursing education programme based on the Cassel Hospital course. There were striking similarities between the Austen Riggs Center and the Cassel Hospital in terms of their history and focus of treatment. Both had been established as private institutions in 1919, and had evolved programmes to serve people with emotional difficulties, using individual psychoanalytically-orientated psychotherapy as the primary mode of treatment. Both were housed in beautiful old estates, with lush grounds, and were relatively small (about 60 beds). They were open facilities; there were no locked doors or coercive restrictions, and the use of medication was limited. Both emphasized the importance of the human relationship as a healing modality, within the context of a therapeutic community, and both were internationally known as teaching and research facilities. There had also been an earlier association between the two institutions, in that Tom Main (then

Medical Director of the Cassel Hospital) had been a visiting scholar at Austen Riggs in 1952.

If the similarities between the two hospitals were striking, so were the differences, many of which had to do with the nurse's role, and how nurses and patients were expected to participate in the therapeutic community programme. At the time of my arrival, the Austen Riggs Center was in the throes of adapting to accommodate more disturbed patients and, therefore, was struggling to balance the needs of the therapeutic community programme with the needs of these individuals for care and attention. Inevitably, this struggle was being played out by the people most intimately involved: the patients and the nursing staff. The Austen Riggs Center was in a similar situation to that of the Cassel Hospital 30 years earlier, when Tom Main, Doreen Weddell (then Matron) and a core group of nurses began the series of study groups that led to the major development of psychosocial nursing (Main, 1968; Weddell, 1968).

Defining the nurse's role: the need for review

As I embarked on a mission to introduce psychosocial nursing at the Austen Riggs Center, it became obvious that the nurse's role needed to be reviewed. It was clear who the patients were, and why they were there. It was not at all clear what the nursing staff's role was, and there were varying and conflicting views on what it should be. Marshall Edelson (1970), in describing the evolution of the community programme at Austen Riggs, had observed the ambiguity of roles and the lack of clear authority, and noted that the nurses themselves were unhappy and unclear about their task priorities. One section of his book was entitled 'No One is Happy with the Nursing Staff'. This was still the case when I arrived.

Whenever we attempt to change something in an organization, it is important to understand its history. My first focus in the review was, therefore, to understand how nursing had developed at Austen Riggs, what values were held, and what was required by people in all parts of the system. We recognized that nursing had evolved from a 'private duty' model: in the early days of the Center, if a patient was particularly disturbed or 'needy', he or she could hire a private duty nurse who was responsible for caring solely for that individual. It might even be that the nurse would accompany the patient after discharge. Nurses still tended to care for individual patients in distress, and there was considerable competition among the patients for this individual attention. The nurses were not confident about how to address the competition other than to endure it.

When the therapeutic community programme was developed during the 1960s, it emphasized a patient-participatory form of self-government, but what was *not* defined was the nurse's role. Without particular training in how to understand and participate in therapeutic groups, only those nurses with a natural affinity or interest in the groups participated in them. Medical staff were appointed as consultants to the groups, so they, unlike the nurses, had a clear role within the therapeutic milieu.

Clarifying the nurse's role involved many hours of meetings to try to formulate and articulate what nurses were doing and why. However, it had also been on my agenda to change what the nurse's role was – to expand it – to do which required demonstrating a broader range of behaviours and possibilities.

Sometimes, what is seen as resistance to change may arise from the fact that people cannot see how else things might be. When this is the case, role models are useful. I had, of course, been talking about Cassel Hospital since I arrived, but I realized that the way I behaved would demonstrate most clearly the ideas I wanted to promote. Whether in groups with patients or staff, I emphasized the nurse's role as participating actively alongside patients in the day-to-day life of the community.

Change through seminar training

The nurse seminar programme at the Cassel provided a starting point for developing a training programme for nurses at the Austen Riggs Center. In these small study groups, we examined nurses' experiences with patients, both from the perspective of what we might learn about patients and from what we might learn about ourselves, and also about how groups function. By using a small group format, we encouraged open communication, trust and co-operation between nurses, thus promoting a more effective team. The examination of our reaction to the patients required, at times, painful reflection on our own feelings, including facing our limitations and fears.

Marilyn Ferguson's now classic book *The Aquarian Conspiracy* (1980) notes that there are four basic ways in which we change when we obtain new and conflicting information. The easiest and most limited of these is *change by exception*; the old belief system remains intact but allows for a handful of anomalies. In *incremental change*, change occurs bit by bit, and the individual is not aware of having changed. In *pendulum change*, there is the abandonment of one closed and certain system for another. The fourth way is *paradigm change*, where a new perspective allows information to come together in a new form or structure. Paradigm change refines and integrates; it absorbs, enlarges and enriches. In paradigm change, we realize that what we know now is only part of what we will know later, and so change is no longer threatening.

Change through exchange

It seemed that incremental change was occurring, but it was paradigm change that I wanted to support. I thought that to encourage this, more role models were needed. In this way, the idea arose of an exchange programme with the Cassel Hospital. The details of the exchange, as they evolved, were that one nurse from Austen Riggs would go to the Cassel Hospital for three or four months, and at the same time a nurse from the Cassel Hospital would come to Austen Riggs. Each hospital continued to pay its own nurse's salary, thus simplifying issues of work visas, licensure, and so on. Each hospital agreed to arrange for housing of the visiting nurse. The visiting nurse worked as a member of an inpatient unit, and was assigned a case-load of patients.

If change is to be effective, people who will be affected, in all parts of the system, need to be involved in the planning. Organizing the exchange programme meant talking about it to many people, to the nurses, the patients, the medical and administrative staff, the activities staff, and anyone else who would be affected by it in any way. While all this talk felt tedious at times, it was, in fact, a crucial part of the exchange programme. We were continually addressing the issue of the nurses' roles and functions, raising the possibility of expanding those roles, and advocating the provision of something more useful to patients. Every time we encountered objections or concerns, there was an opportunity to explore people's fears, and to consider aspects that might not otherwise be addressed.

The outcome

There were three exchanges during the four years from 1978 to 1981. The programme accomplished what we had hoped for: to provide a working model of how to practise psychosocial nursing, adapted to the Austen

Riggs setting at that time. As a direct result of the first exchange, we changed the structure of the nurse–patient working relationship to a primary nursing model, from what had been a more diffuse method of team nursing. In primary nursing, each patient is assigned a particular nurse who is primarily responsible for co-ordinating that patient's care, including ongoing collaboration with the patient's psychotherapist.

Each exchange nurse was encouraged to take on a project which could be completed within the three months' visit. The first nurse to come to us from the Cassel Hospital, Claire Haidon, developed a questionnaire about the nursing role, which was distributed to therapists, nurses and patients. When the results were presented back to them, a lively discussion ensued.

Janet Rooney was the first nurse to go from the Austen Riggs Center to the Cassel Hospital. When she returned, she took on a decorating project with patients to refurbish a particularly gloomy TV room. There was some surprise that nurses and patients were doing what was normally considered to be a task for the maintenance department, but numerous other projects evolved from this beginning. Eventually, a decorating committee came to be an accepted part of the community programme. This committee, which included patients, nurses and administrative staff, reviewed requests and allocated monies for patient–nurse-initiated activities. Such activities were increasingly recognized for their therapeutic potential; they helped to reinforce the healthy capacities of patients rather than encourage regression and dependency in the hospital setting.

In order to maximize the impact of this work, each of the Austen Riggs Center nurses, when they returned from the Cassel Hospital, took on the role of community nurse. In this role, they had responsibility for working with the community as a whole, expanding and developing the nursing presence in the community programme. By the time Janet became the head nurse, her Cassel perspective was accepted as the norm for nursing at the Austen Riggs Center.

The second exchange nurse from the Cassel Hospital was Mic Rafferty. He developed a course to prepare the most experienced nurses to sit the American Nurses' Association Certification Examination in Psychiatric-Mental Health Nursing. The course included a training in leadership and supervisory skills.

At the Cassel Hospital, the collaborative working relationship of the doctor and the nurse is supported by a meeting structure which aims to facilitate open and honest communication. At the Austen Riggs Center, this relationship had been less valued, but one significant outcome of the nurse exchange programme was to highlight this discrepancy, and to work deliberately toward changing it. As nurses became clearer about their own realm of practice, and felt empowered and supported in doing their work, they talked about it in meetings with doctors, and a closer collaboration evolved.

When we, as change agents, plant an idea from one system to another, conditions in the system we are attempting to change will influence and shape both the final outcome and each step of the process. The attitude with which we undertake change is important and needs to be respectful and positive. Change cannot be coerced or dictated from above. When we meet with resistance to change, we need to work with it, even welcome it, for the perspective it brings to the process. Finally, it is important not to be too heavily invested in any particular outcome. When not constricted, movement is towards growth, and a system will evolve its own solutions when encouraged by an atmosphere of respect and trust.

Acknowledgements

I would like to acknowledge and thank each of the nurses who participated in the nurse exchange programme: Janet Rooney, Claire Haidon, Mary Kate Thompson, Mic Rafferty, Nancy Peck and Alf Bowers. Thanks also to Louise de Lambert, Senior Nursing Officer at the Cassel Hospital, and to Edith Breed, Director of Nursing at the Austen Riggs Center, for their support of this project.

References

Edelson, M. (1970). *The Practice of Sociotherapy: A Case Study.* Yale University Press.
Ferguson, M. (1980). *The Aquarian Conspiracy,* pp. 71–72, Tarcher.
Main, T.F. (1968). The ailment. In *Psychosocial Nursing: Studies from the Cassel Hospital* (E. Barnes, ed.) pp. 33–60, Tavistock Publications.
Weddell, D. (1968). Change as a learning situation. In *Psychosocial Nursing: Studies from the Cassel Hospital* (E. Barnes, ed.) pp. 299–303, Tavistock Publications.

Chapter 4

National policy and professional practice

Gillian Chapman

Working in a therapeutic community such as the Cassel Hospital has similarities to working as a civil servant in the Department of Health. In a therapeutic community, in working with other team members the aim is to create an environment in which care can be given and in which the opportunities for patients to function are maximized. Words, particularly spoken words, are a prime means by which this is undertaken. The way that words are used by nurses in a therapeutic community is informed by a range of theories of human behaviour (Chapman, 1988a, 1988b), but what predominates, when all else fails, is recourse to common-sense reasoning.

When working as a civil servant in a state department, as a member of the team, and with the agreement of ministers, words, particularly written words, are used to explain and implement the government policies that determine the environment in which care takes place nationally. The way in which these words are used is informed by implicit understanding about the nature of democracy. Both parliamentary democracy and therapeutic communities thrive on the use of language, underpinned by rational or theoretical principles, the practical applications of which inform the use and understanding of the words used.

Moodie (1984), for example, believes that governing is about the process of making rules by which social, economic and cultural conduct can be regulated. Language, whether used to gain insight and to remedy personal difficulties, or to find solutions to social problems, is preferable to the use of force. This chapter explores these issues in more detail and, briefly, describes key policies which are currently influencing nursing practice.

What do civil servants do?

Since the transmission of *Yes, Minister* by the BBC in the 1980s, and the widely published quotation by Sir Robert Armstrong, of being 'economical with the truth', there has been considerable fascination with and possible mistrust of civil servants (Young, and Sloeman, 1982). This is hardly surprising because the civil service is concerned with the conduct of a whole range of government activities which affect the community. Civil servants administrate 'the mechanisms through which governing occurs – rule making and application, policy making and implementation, and they make use of legal and other sanctions to ensure rules and policies are observed' (Chapman, 1992).

What do social scientists say about governing and language?

Sociologists, preoccupied with the use of language in society, have studied the words and texts produced by officials in this country and others. Foucault (1961, 1973, 1977, 1982) concentrated on the way in which our attitudes towards one another and human behaviour emerge in particular historical periods, and are expressed in and through knowledge constructed as discourse. Discourse is the set of ideas, beliefs, theories and dialogues about human beings which become accepted as a valid and objective knowledge in a particular society. He notes that such discourse is used not only to explain human beings and their everyday activities but also to shape professional practice and techniques used in dealing with individuals, both within and outside institutions (Chapman, 1988a, 1988b).

It is interesting to scan official documents, not only for what they say about the government policy of the day but also for the extent to which they reflect or echo professional discourse. This book could be considered in this way.

Key policy issues of relevance to psychosocial nursing

During the last 20 years, many government initiatives have demonstrated concerns for, first, the individudal users, and, secondly, the partnership between client and professional. These include the recent NHS reforms, *Caring for People* (Department of Health, 1989), *The Health of the*

Nation (Department of Health, 1992), *The Patient's Charter* (Department of Health, 1991), *A Vision for the Future* (NHS Management Executive, 1993), and *Working in Partnership* (Department of Health, 1994a). All of these place users of the service and their carers at the centre, and demand that the service be based on an assessment of individual need and offered in partnership with users, their families and carers in an interagency setting which provides high quality and cost-effective care.

The signs are that the Labour administration will continue to stress the importance of this partnership.

A Vision for the Future

The philosophical basis of nursing, midwifery and health visiting is readily adapted to the goals set out in *A Vision for the Future* (NHS Management Executive, 1993). This national strategic framework for the nursing profession takes as given that the professions are concerned with enabling the individual, whether adult or child, and his or her family to achieve and maintain their optimal physical, psychological and social wellbeing when that individual or his or her carers cannot achieve this unaided. It notes:

> The values which flow from these shared activities are essentially concerned with an understanding and appreciation of each patient or client; a fundamental respect for the individual; a respect for the integrity of the individual and the person's right to an honest, and principled response which preserves his or her dignity and facilitates an active participation in care.

The document sets out the contribution that nurses, midwives and health visitors can make to the health of the population and the quality of health care provided by the NHS. In the context of the policies mentioned above, it identifies some key targets and practical ways in which nurses, midwives and health visitors can contribute to the delivery of high quality, cost-effective health care. Nurses at the Cassel Hospital will be familiar with the principles in these strategic aims and objectives:

- To work with colleagues towards common goals, focusing on patients' and clients' needs;
- Encouraging participation of the users of the service and their carers in partnership with other professionals and agencies;
- Contributing to improvements in the general health of the population of England;
- Ensuring a high quality, cost-effective service.

A Vision for the Future has five main objectives:

- *Accountability for practice:* developing a clear understanding of the responsibilities and obligations associated with individual professional accountability;
- *Quality, outcomes and audit:* providing high quality, cost-effective care based on the assessment of individual needs, with nurses', midwives' and health visitors' interventions evaluated, outcomes charted and the results submitted to professional audit;
- *Clinical and professional leadership, research and supervision:* providing credible clinical and professional leadership as part of the corporate management agenda;
- *Purchasing:* ensuring that clinical and professional expertise feeds into the purchasing and commissioning cycle;
- *Education and personal development:* recognising and promoting the educational and personal development needs of nurses, midwives and health visitors as an integral part of the delivery of high quality health care.

Twelve targets for action were identified from these five objectives. Many of the targets fit very neatly with the philosophy developed at the Cassel Hospital over many years. Examples of these targets include: assigning each patient/client to a named nurse, midwife or health visitor, throughout the period of care; surveying the quality of the partnership with users and their involvement in care; taking steps to discuss with each professional how they might develop their practice; encouraging care that is specific to the individual needs of patients; and looking at the appropriateness of clinical supervision as a means of improving quality care.

Developments in *A Vision for the Future* are set out in an executive letter and report from the Chief Nursing Officer (Department of Health, 1995 (13)) as is the concept of clinical supervision (Department of Health, 1994b (5)).

Working in Partnership

Working in Partnership: a Collaborative Approach to Care (Department of Health, 1994a), the report of the Mental Health Nursing Review Team, notes that the first official review of mental health nursing, *Psychiatric Nursing Today and Tomorrow* (Ministry of Health, 1968) focused on inpatient psychiatric nursing. *Working in Partnership* is the second. It was commissioned by the Secretary of State to reflect on developments since 1968, including: changes in the legal framework; shifts in social, political and economic policy; alterations in public attitudes and expectations; and the move towards a more individualized approach to care.

Many of the recommendations would be very familiar to nurses at the Cassel Hospital, who would also feel considerable sympathy for the approach taken, that the work of mental health nurses rests on their relationship with the people who use the service and that they should focus their skills on those with acute and enduring mental illness. The report states that to be effective this relationship should have value to both partners, the nurse and the client.

The review made 42 recommendations. The skills it suggests that mental health nurses should have are worth restating, while acknowledging other members of the professional team operate from a related knowledge and skills base, the review team emphasizes the unique contribution of mental health nurses:

- Establish a therapeutic relationship which rests on a respect for others and a skilled therapeutic use of self;
- Sustain such relationships over time and respond flexibly to the changing needs of those with mental health problems;
- Construct, implement and evaluate a care programme;
- Provide skilled assessment and on-going monitoring;
- Make risk assessments and judgements;
- Monitor the dosage, effects and contra-indications of medication;
- Detect early signs of deteriorating mental health, including potential self-harm and suicide risk, worsening physical condition and potential threats to others;
- Prioritize work in order to respond to those most in need;
- Collaborate with all members of the multidisciplinary team;
- Network effectively, setting appropriate boundaries to professional input;
- Manage the therapeutic environment, determined by clear awareness of issues such as safety, dignity and partnership.

As a manifesto of commitment, these principles should be familiar to nurses working in a psychosocial environment.

The team also identified what they considered to be the characteristics of the best models of mental health nursing practice, as shown below.

The Cassel Hospital has provided a good example of this type of practice for many years:

- A clearly informed assessment of client needs, which involves the clients and their carers;
- An understanding of the needs and perceptions of the local community and positive efforts to promote awareness;
- A conscious effort to deal sensitively with issues of race, creed and gender;
- Full and open collaboration with others, including colleagues from other professions, other nurses, midwives and health visitors, and non-professional helpers;
- Accessibility and flexibility of managers;
- Identification of very clear objectives for intervention, clear measures of outcome and means of performance review;
- The provision of high quality managerial support for the mental health nurse, together with constant access to clinical supervision and continued professional development.

Partnerships with patients

Patient Partnership: Building a Collaborative Strategy, published by the Department of Health, NHS Management Executive, stresses the importance of putting patients first and of ensuring that health services and care are truly responsive to the needs of users and patients. It acknowledges that there is always scope to do more to identify and spread best practice, to develop and apply a proper evidence base, and to ensure that organizational, cultural and resource constraints are identified and addressed.

The aim of the *Patient Partnership* strategy is as follows: at the level of individual patient care, to promote users' involvement in their own care as active partners with professionals and enable patients to become informed about their treatment and care, and to make informed decisions and choices about these if they wish; and, at the level of overall service development, to contribute to the quality of health services by making them more responsive to the needs and preferences of users, and ensure that users have the knowledge, skills and support to enable them to influence NHS service policy and planning.

This document acknowledges the profession's commitment throughout the NHS in emphasizing communication skills and working in partnership with patients. It stresses the importance of supporting staff in achieving active partnership and user involvement, noting that there are complex and sensitive issues where the professions, management and patient groups all have a role to play in learning from each other:

> If patient partnership is to succeed it will require the long term commitment of all health service staff. There is often no fundamental unwillingness to involve patients on the part of managers or professionals, but there are real issues and challenges to be addressed. As with any other group that deals with the public, some NHS staff will, for a variety of reasons, have problems with the very difficult task of communicating effectively and sensitively. The notion of partnership can be unsettling. It raises difficult issues about where professional responsibilities begin and end. Some would argue that such a change could make jobs more difficult by creating more demanding patients.

The document notes that, while there is a range of activities seeking to involve patients within the NHS, there is no consolidated, reviewed body of knowledge about techniques that are most appropriate and the circumstances in which they should be used. It is here, surely, that organizations that share a culture of developing relationships with patients through the use of words and reflection have much to contribute, both in terms of a body of knowledge and of the techniques by which understandings derived from it are shared with individuals and groups. Organizations such as the Cassel Hospital, preoccupied as they are with involving patients in a therapeutic partnership, have much to say and share with other organizations on how to go about creating a culture that will enable sensitive, continuing therapeutic conversations and relationships between patients and professionals about the problems that bother them and the means by which these problems might be resolved.

Conclusion

In conclusion, there are clear links between the work of the therapeutic community, with its preoccupation with words and the liberating power of understanding through talk, and theories about the nature of language and discourse. This chapter suggests implicitly that, to the extent that the therapeutic community is an element of the society in which it exists and that society is governed by means of a democratic process, there will be echoes and reflections of therapeutic philosophies and discourses in government policies about the care of patients. The highlighting of key government department policy documents traces those aspects of policy with which nurses working in therapeutic communities might feel a sense of recognition and ease.

References

Chapman, G.E. (1988a). Text talk and discourse in a therapeutic community. *Int. J. Ther. Communities*, **9**(2), 75–87.

Chapman, G.E. (1988b). Reporting therapeutic discourse in a therapeutic community. *J. Adv. Nurs.*, **13**, 255–264.

Chapman, G.E. (1992). Politics power and psychiatric nursing. In *A Textbook of Psychiatric and Mental Health Nursing* (J. Brooking, S. Ritter and B. Thamas, eds.) pp. 507–517.

Department of Health. (1989). *Caring for People: Community Care in the Next Decade and Beyond*. HMSO.

Department of Health. (1991). *The Patient's Charter*. HMSO.

Department of Health. (1992). *The Health of the Nation: a Strategy for Health in England and Wales*. HMSO.

Department of Health. (1994a). *Working in Partnership: a Collaborative Approach to Care*. (A report of the Mental Health Nursing Review Team.).

Department of Health. (1994b). Chief Nursing Officer Letter(5): *Clinical Supervision*.

Department of Health. (1996). *Patient Partnership: Building a Collaborative Strategy*.

Foucault, M. (1961). *Madness and Civilisation*. Fontana.

Foucault, M. (1973). *The Birth of the Clinic*. Tavistock Publications.

Foucault, M. (1977). *Discipline and Punish*. Penguin.

Foucault, M. (1982). The subject and power. *Crit. Inquiry.* **8**, 778–795.

Ministry of Health. (1968). *Psychiatric Nursing Today and Tomorrow*. (Standing Mental Health and Standing Nursing Advisory Committees.)

Moodie, G.C. (1984). Politics is about government. In *What is Politics?* (A. Leftwich, ed.) pp. 19–33, Blackwell.

NHS Management Executive. (1993). *A Vision for the Future: the Nursing, Midwifery and Health Visiting Contribution to Health and Health Care*.

Young, H. and Sloeman, A. (1982). *No Minister: an Enquiry into the Civil Service*. BBC Publications.

Section Two

Practice

Introduction

Jacqueline Ord

The emphasis in this section is on putting psychosocial principles into practice. The six authors show how psychosocial practice is informed by the theories outlined in Section One, and is supported by professional development, as described in Section Three. They write from a variety of perspectives: from nursing at the Cassel Hospital, to nursing in the community; and from social work to psychotherapy to general nursing.

Graham McCaffrey's chapter, 'The use of leisure activities in psychosocial nursing', gives a picture of what it is like to work as part of the community team at the Cassel Hospital. He describes the context in which nurses and patients work together, and the structures through which shared activities are integrated into the therapeutic programme. This provides a rich environment for patients to develop their capacities for working and playing together, and for taking responsibility for themselves and each other. Fritha Irwin describes her work, also within the Cassel Hospital, with a young woman, Hannah, who's sense of self and whose trust in others had been shattered. In 'Nursing an adult survivor of childhood sexual abuse', she gives a personal account of the sometimes very frightening and difficult relationship she had with this young woman, and how this relationship helped Hannah to grow beyond her abuse, to find new ways of relating to others.

Vicky Mills' chapter, 'The use of self in child protection work', describes her work with families where children are at risk. In her role as social worker, and working within legislative frameworks that can make the task very difficult, she draws on the knowledge of psychodynamic processes which she developed during her nurse training at the Cassel Hospital. This knowledge helps her to tolerate and work with the processes that operate within dysfunctional families, and also within the teams that work with them. It also helps her to go on learning, as she illustrates through her example of her five years' work with Mona and her children, an experience which she describes as an 'emotional roller coaster'.

Ann Simpson, in 'Mary's story', writes from the perspective of a nurse who trained at the Cassel Hospital, but is now working with families in the community. She demonstrates, through her work with Mary and her family, how psychosocial principles can be transferred into the community setting. In the process, we obtain a vivid picture of Mary, herself a survivor of childhood abuse, and her efforts, together with her husband, to create a better physical and emotional environment for themselves and their children. Ann's nursing, informed by psychodynamic understanding, and supported by her colleagues, plays an important part in their improvement. Just when things seem to be going well, however, the family have to deal with the terrible news that Mary has developed a fatal illness. How they deal with this illness is a tribute to the courage of Mary, her family and their nurse.

Gillian Parker writes as a Cassel nurse who has for many years practised as a psychotherapist. In 'Pain as memory', she explores the deep connections between body and mind, to show the consequences for the victim of abuse which is too terrible to remember or to talk about. She illustrates, through examples of her work with people who have suffered 'soul murder' the ways in which physical symptoms and unspeakable emotional damage are linked. She shows the importance of creating a holding structure within which patients can feel safe enough to remember and talk about their abuse. These understandings have profound importance for nurses and others whose care encompasses the patient as whole person, including body, mind and history.

Finally, in this section, Louise de Raeve raises some thought-provoking questions in her chapter, 'Knowing patients: how much and how well?' She brings a subtle and searching philosophical perspective to aspects of knowing patients that nurses often take for granted, and raises issues that are of vital concern, not only for general nurses but for practitioners in all disciplines. In the process, she explores the importance of respecting the emotional, as well as the physical, boundaries of the people in our care, and the need to help patients to guard themselves against possible intrusions by well-meaning professionals.

Chapter 5
The use of leisure activities in psychosocial nursing

Graham McCaffrey

In this chapter, I explore the use of social and leisure activities as part of the therapeutic programme of the Cassel Hospital. In order to establish the context, there is a brief introduction to the principles of the therapeutic community and the nurse's role at the Cassel Hospital. The structures are described by which social and leisure activities within the hospital are integrated into the therapeutic work. Some of the therapeutic opportunities that arise when nurses work alongside patients in the course of such activities are included. There is a discussion of the significance of the voluntary element in this area of practice and the related problems for both nurses and patients.

The hospital uses a treatment model somewhat different from that of most other therapeutic communities, but it shares with them some essential attributes as described by Kennard (1983). These are:

1. An informal and communal atmosphere;
2. The central place of group meetings in the therapeutic programme;
3. Sharing the work of maintaining and running the community;
4. The recognition of patients or residents as auxiliary therapists, commenting on and influencing each other's behaviour and attitudes;
5. A motivating belief in the value of psychodynamic processes as agents for enquiry and personal change.

Nursing work: model of intervention

The patients admitted for this mode of treatment are severely disturbed. They invariably have a history of trauma in their early development, often of sexual abuse. As adults or adolescents they have exhibited disturbance which has adversely affected one or more aspects of their life to an extreme degree and this is manifest in the ways they relate to others. A patient might, for example, respond to intensive feelings of frustration or anger by resorting to compulsive self-harming behaviour. Self-mutilation, binge drinking, bulimia and taking overdoses are all forms of behaviour commonly encountered.

Nurses have a central role, working with patients through facilitating groups, doing practical tasks, and running many community functions alongside them. Patients are involved by co-managing aspects of community life with nurses. These include the ordering of food, arranging rotas for cooking, cleaning, and responding to patients who appear very distressed or at risk of harming themselves or others. In the course of this close work with patients, nurses develop an awareness of patients' difficulties, as they emerge.

A patient in a daily cleaning group, for example, took on more and more of the work, cleaning the kitchen excessively but not allowing others to share responsibility. This was questioned and discussed by nurses both while it was happening and in subsequent community meetings. This enabled the patient to re-examine her behaviour and talk about her fear of losing control over feelings of anger and despair, which she was driving away through frantic activity. This process helped her to come to a more mutual, shared approach towards working with others.

Nursing interventions and outcomes are assessed by peer group discussion and co-ordinated with the patient's psychotherapist in the multidisciplinary team. Through the use of knowledge and understanding gained as a result of such interactions, nurses attempt to formulate collaborative individual treatment plans with patients. One dimension of the nursing approach is to express spontaneous and honest emotional responses to patients. This always has to be tempered by judgements about what is professionally appropriate and by the therapeutic need, always leaving open a space for further dialogue with patients. This approach incorporates a notion of normative social and emotional expectations (for example: that people turn up to do a job they have agreed to do unless they have given a good reason not to; or that shock, upset and anger are realistic responses to the sight of self-inflicted wounds). The idea of the normative in the community also incorporates some individual variation, so that, although nurses share a common core approach, they do not adhere to a uniform set of ideas and responses. The emphasis on socially normative routines, activities and behaviours supports a manifest conceptualization of the therapeutic community as a microcosm of its surrounding society, but it is an environment that is contained and, to a degree, protected, in order to allow patients, many of whom have severe difficulties, to cope with an emotionally-testing and anxiety-provoking treatment.

Activities: definition and clinical context

The use of activities is one part of nurses' work. The term 'activities' denotes one particular segment of the social microcosm, namely, voluntary, social, leisure activities. There are a number of reasons why activities are accorded a high value and importance within the therapeutic programme. In the social microcosm aspect of a therapeutic community, they simply form part of a normative idea that a balanced and satisfactory life involves both work and leisure. Patients invariably have difficulties in both of these aspects of social life. Beyond this, because the community also requires enquiry and self-reflection about feelings and behaviour, it is also important to work out a thoroughgoing rationale for activities in order that patients and staff can see how they can become an active element in therapeutic work.

The word 'activities' describes things that people might ordinarily do in the space of leisure time outside their working hours. These include: cultural activities such as painting, going to the theatre or reading poetry; sport and exercise such as badminton, aerobics and swimming; and indoor games such as chess, pool and table tennis. My own clinical experience was of organizing, with a patient, a poetry reading group.

Activities in the hospital are not exactly the same as those people do in leisure time at home. In the hospital, leisure must have active, social and managed elements. Watching television, for example, takes up a large part of many people's free time but it is not an activity within the therapeutic programme. By a fine distinction, however, there is a video activity. The difference is that the selection and showing of a video film requires an individual to take some responsibility to make a choice of film, negotiate and maintain the boundaries of time and venue, and try to drum up some interest in a shared experience.

The element of choice within this activity became a focus for clinical work with an adolescent patient who took on the job of managing the video activity. He was very socially withdrawn and inexpressive, yet harboured violent fantasies by which he sometimes felt troubled. He undermined the principle of working with a nurse by arranging video viewing nights at times other than those agreed. In addition, he rented films with a violent content, without consulting anyone else, which were disturbing to some other patients. Thus, his involvement with the activity had distinct social implications, which provided a source of therapeutic work. His behaviour was questioned by nurses and by other patients, encouraging him to think about possible connections between his private fantasies and his actions in the social world of the hospital. The social dimension of activities is, therefore, one of the keys to their therapeutic usefulness in meeting the needs of individual patients and in providing points of therapeutic intervention.

Organizational context

The distinction between what is and is not an activity becomes clearer when it is placed in the context of the therapeutic community's structures. The hospital (unlike most therapeutic communities) has all sorts of subdivisions within it. It is divided into three units, for single adults, families and adolescents. There is also a division of labour between the psychotherapists, who see patients for individual and group psychotherapy, and the nurses, who participate in everyday work such as cooking, cleaning and leisure activities. Patients might choose to talk about activities in a therapy session, but primarily these discussions come within the sphere of the nursing work.

Leisure activities are part of the remit of the community team, which administers the supraunit aspects of the therapeutic community. In other words, activities are open to patients from all of the units and can provide opportunities for working with a wider range of people. The activities are overseen by a committee of patients elected by themselves. The committee consists of a chairperson, treasurer and secretary; they work with one of the two nurses from the community team. There is no fixed term for committee members to serve. They usually continue in one of the jobs for about three months, trying to keep in mind its relevance and usefulness in pursuing their individual treatment aims. For example, an aim might be to look at a patient's pattern of avoidance of regular responsibility, or to encourage him or her to explore the value of social activities if the patient has been very isolated.

The activities chairperson chairs the weekly activities meeting and also attends a weekly meeting in which other senior staff and patient representatives discuss issues affecting the community. This latter function reflects the importance attached to the state of activities within the hospital. The wish and capacity of patients to be together and to do things voluntarily together, or its opposite extreme, social isolationism, can be used as a measure of the social cohesion, or of the level of disturbance, within the patient group.

The secretary takes minutes of the weekly meeting, types them and presents copies at the next meeting. These tasks might appear mundane, but they can offer openings for therapeutic nursing work. At a level of basic skills, patients with poor literacy have used the job of secretary to practise listening and writing skills. With careful attention from a nurse, the job offers a venue where anxiety and feelings of shame about poor literacy skills can be shared, worked upon, and, thereby, reduced.

At a more complex emotional level, one young woman doing the secretary's job regularly failed to present the minutes. She either did not write them at all, or destroyed the finished copy before the weekly meeting. Observation of this pattern by the activities nurse led to it being discussed among the committee. It emerged that the patient had such a fear of any error being seen by others, that she would avoid presenting her minutes to the meeting. It was then arranged that one other patient, with whom she felt safe, would look at the minutes with her and reassure her about her work, which, in reality, was of a high standard. Once this plan was implemented, the patient was able, with increasing confidence, to present the minutes and test out her anxiety against the reality that other people were more interested in using the minutes in the meeting, than in scouring them for minor mistakes.

The treasurer keeps track of the annual budget for activities and of a weekly fund for sundries such as newspapers. Decisions about funding requests are made by the whole committee and by the nurse working with them, who is ultimately responsible for the budget.

The therapeutic possibilities arise from a patient undertaking the secretary's or the treasurer's role. For example, issues of budgeting, trust and giving to others may take on a specific meaning and usage to individual patients.

The weekly activities meeting, convened by the committee, the nurse and the community doctor, is open to all patients and nurses. People usually attend because they manage an activity. Each activity is run by a nurse and a patient manager. It is up to them to initiate the activity, to establish a time and a venue for it, and to make requests for any funding they think they may need. Money can be used for anything from a new table tennis ball to theatre tickets, or from pottery clay to purchasing CDs.

Social and therapeutic purpose

Different categories of activity can present scope for work with the problems that patients may have in particular areas of functioning. Activities can have positive attributes and countervailing psychological obstacles. I offer three examples.

Physical activities

Swimming and exercise improve fitness and provide a sense of physical wellbeing. They can enhance confidence through learning and demonstrating a skill that gives a sense of physical freedom and co-ordination.

However, there is also an emotional domain which can be acknowledged by the nurse in talking with patients about their experience of such activities, and in sharing their own feelings and attitudes towards their own bodies and/or their feelings about other people's bodies. For example, if a patient bears scars from self-mutilation, undressing to go swimming might help that individual to face up to other people's reaction to his or her behaviour.

A patient who had a long history of anorexia and who exercised excessively to burn off calories, wished to manage an aerobics activity. There was open discussion about the advisability of this for her, with conflicting opinions expressed among the staff team. In the end, the activity went ahead with the aim of performing relatively gentle exercises. The patient's primary nurse monitored her weight with her to ensure that it did not fall below a medically determined minimum level. The possibility of a harmful effect of the activity was thus kept in balance against the social and fitness benefits it provided at the same time.

Poetry reading

This allows one, literally, to speak out. It calls into play an appreciation of language, rhythm, critical intelligence and personal taste. It is a venue for an imaginative freedom in response to emotionally charged language, which can, at times, feel exposing. Difficulties can be explored in sessions with the patient's therapist, which include anxiety about revealing something of one's inner emotional world, and anxiety about performing in front of others.

The first patient manager of the poetry reading group used the emotional force present in poetry to memorable effect. He kicked off the opening meeting of the group by reading Larkin's (1974) poem *This be the Verse*, which begins: 'They fuck you up, your mum and dad.' He took the opportunity, appropriately, to use something that gave vent to a feeling of his own.

A later patient manager of the group was preoccupied with Byronic fantasies about her nurse co-manager. As a result, she tried to exclude other patients from the group. Her wish to let fantasy push out the reality of her role, as a group leader, had to be tactfully pointed out. This example raises again the crucial interpersonal and social aspect of activities. For this patient, the episode brought up questions about her previous social isolation and why she feared and resented social contact outside the comfortable illusion of an imagined intimacy.

Bicycle maintenance

This requires dexterity and technical skill, which includes a conscientiousness about finishing a job properly. It tests the intrapsychic reparative capacity of an individual by means of carrying out an actual repair to a machine. Jaques (1960) describes this as an element in all work.

Emergence of self in relation to others through activities

A useful dimension in all kinds of activities is the taking of pride in one's talents and the capacity to allow others to see them. For people with low self-esteem, this can be a difficult but valuable thing to achieve. It entails distinguishing oneself within, or from, the group of patients and, thereby, risking losing a place within it. This means potentially having to overcome the safe but often stifling inertia of the pseudomutual group (Gustafson, 1976), which pretends there are no differences within it, in order to maintain a false stability. I observed this happening in the poetry group, with a patient manager who struggled to work with me in making any decisions, for example, about which new books to buy. She tried continually to involve the rest of the group in order to avoid distinguishing herself as the designated patient manager.

Another component of activities is the ability to play. This is an important part of childhood development. When such development has been impaired, an adult can find it painfully difficult to relax, have fun and be playful. The community's activities offer a series of spaces in which to play in a safe environment. The idea of play can be extended to include an element in creative tasks such as painting or sculpting. These have a laborious and serious side to them, but they also require a playfulness in the sense of being able to imagine disparate elements transformed into a new whole. This is equivalent to the component of work which Jaques calls 'lysis and scanning'. There must be a plasticity in the mental process to synthesize the available conscious and unconscious elements pertaining to a task. If, however, 'the mental process is concrete and inflexible, the bits and particles are not available for synthesis' (Jaques, 1960) and no new integration of elements can emerge.

Activities enable people to encounter each other in ways different from those determined by their usual work roles. This happens in patient–patient interactions but even more so in patient–nurse interactions. An extreme example is the hospital's annual Christmas revue, written and performed by nurses and patients together. This invariably includes some satirical digs at the institution, and permits patients and nurses to dress up and act together in outrageous characterizations. There is often a literal role reversal, with patients taking the part of nurses and vice versa. Participants on either side are able to express some of the things they envy, are jealous of, dislike or are amused by in the other. These, of course, are secrets to no one, but are usually only tacitly understood. Nurses can act out their jealousy of what they sometimes experience as the patient's freedom to refuse to join in community life; conversely, patients can adopt the persona of the nurse who, as they sometimes experience, is always in the right.

To a lesser degree, this experience of seeing oneself and others differently is present in all activities. For example, in the morning meeting, a nurse might be battling with a patient to try to get him to talk about why he had not helped to cook supper the night before; in the afternoon, the same nurse and patient could be battling it out in a game of table tennis. These are quite different moments for each participant in the same relationship. The nurturing of such experiences provides patients (and nurses) with the possibility of seeing different parts of others and oneself, and leads to the toleration and appreciation of diversity in relationships. The development of opportunities for such experiences is at the core of psychosocial nursing.

Voluntary space

A crucial point about activities, which underpins all the other considerations, is that they make use of voluntary space. In the social analogy, this is free time, as opposed to work time, or as Mark Twain (1976) puts it in Tom Sawyer; 'Work consists of whatever a body is obliged to do, and play consists of whatever a body is not obliged to do'. The voluntary nature of activities lends them an important dimension, as part of treatment. Jaques (1960) discusses the ego strength that is required to perform a task, in order to bear the uncertainty of its outcome and to contain the intrapsychic and real separating out and reintegration of parts of a task.

In most parts of the therapeutic programme, there is an institutional obligation to perform a task. The rota to cook supper for the community, for example, carries considerable weight in the community, and peer pressure among patients is the main instrument of its enforcement. In this case, there is a powerful external containment (in the form of the peer pressure) for processing the task. In contrast, in activities, there is far less external containment and the consequences of failure to carry out a task are far less severe. The badminton activity not taking place will have far less impact on the community than the supper not being cooked. It may be argued, therefore, that activities can offer more of a testing ground of a patient's capacity to work in Jaques' sense. The performance of the task is less bounded and supported by external structures and, consequently, is more dependent on the patient's own, internal, ego-strength.

In practice, patient and nurse co-managers will encourage their peers to join in an activity, say a game of football. The co-managers invariably feel an emotional investment in the game being successful because they have provided an impetus and wish for it to happen. The significance of egostrength operating in voluntary space applies particularly to the individuals in this situation. In arranging the game, they have summoned up internal psychological resources, such as the capacity to hold to the idea of a successful realization of the wished-for game. In doing this, they have been able to contain their fears that no one else will want to play and that they will feel rejected, or that people will play but not enjoy themselves and that they will feel resented. If an unconscious destructive urge on the managers' part has not got in the way, they will also have assembled the physical resource of ball, field and goalposts. When such efforts are undertaken out of one's own wishes and imagination, and not because one has been told to undertake them, there is a self-affirming quality (even if the activity was only partially successful). Patients' involvement in voluntary activities can stimulate the inherent potential, for feelings of self-worth and pleasure, which can be difficult to reach in more formalized areas of clinical work.

In the hospital, there is a discernible cycle in activities, a period of enthusiasm followed by one of disillusionment and apathy. The task falls to the managers of the activity, both nurse and patient, either to look for ways of sustaining it and trying to reawaken interest, or to let it slide into disuse and end it. Many objective factors influence the outcome, for example, whether the patient is soon to leave the hospital, or either the patient's or the nurse manager's other commitments. Even the time of year can be important if it is a seasonal sport. It is, however, also a question, at such times, of the degree of value and commitment they continue to attach to the activity when they know they do not have to take part in it.

However, the notion of voluntary space in a therapeutic community is problematic and the analogy of leisure time at a certain point can no longer apply. For patients, the inclusiveness of a therapeutic community blurs the line between work and leisure. Leisure activities undoubtedly feel different from other parts of treatment, but they are still done with the same people in the same building and are still subject to the therapeutic eye. This is different from the work/leisure dichotomy, where there are generally much clearer distinctions of time, place and participants between the two.

The complexity is even more marked for nurses. They are encouraged to take on managing and participating in activities for which they feel some personal enthusiasm and yet they also have to do them because it is part of their job. There is a paradox that activities must be voluntary, or an essential point about them is lost, and yet they must be done because they represent an essential part of life, and an obligatory part of the nurse's role.

In practice, this is worked out uneasily. Nurse managers become frustrated with junior nurses if they are not undertaking an activity and nurses struggle perennially to find time to do so. The institution compounds the difficulty by fixing the times and venues of a plethora of meetings. It is difficult to find free spaces in the timetabled day in which to hold activities, since, in this respect, they maintain their voluntary identity. Sometimes they are pushed into 'free' time after the end of the nurse's working day. I used to do this with the poetry reading group, because it was the only way I felt able to concentrate on it and leave my other duties. This indicates the lower priority nurses eventually give to activities as opposed to other parts of their role, and also, I suggest, some ambivalence or confusion about mixing 'work' and 'leisure'.

Conclusion

I have discussed some of the therapeutic possibilities of leisure activities in the nursing of disturbed patients. One recurring theme is the social dimension of activities. They offer a milieu of relating to other people in a freer way than is possible in more task-oriented or role-defined settings. The anxiety engendered by less defined space is offset by the stakes of success and failure being lowered. The possibilities of patients developing a sense of social being within activities counters the social isolation, which has often been a long-established feature of their lives. A second fundamental theme is the possibility of creative self-expression and self-affirmation in all kinds of leisure activity, not only those, such as art and writing, which we automatically think of as creative. This runs counter to the self-destructive forms of expression, which, again, have often long been a pattern of patients' lives.

This chapter looks at activities, in a specialized sense, as part of the psychosocial work of nurses at the Cassel Hospital. This is a specific area, but I believe that wider points for nurses and others can be drawn from it. When rehabilitation is the purpose of care, different tasks may have different social meanings, which can influence the carer–patient relationship and the carer's own attitude to work. Goals in treatment can be related to particular activities, concerning both the social equivalents of activities within the treatment setting and with regard to the tasks involved and their specific therapeutic potential.

References

Gustafson, J.P. (1976). The pseudo-mutual small group or institution. *Hum. Relations*, **29**, 989–997.

Jaques, E. (1960). Disturbances in the capacity to work. *J. Psychoanal.*, **41**, 357–367.

Kennard, D. (1983). *An Introduction to Therapeutic Communities*, pp. 7–8, Routledge.

Larkin, P. (1974). *High Windows*. Faber.

Twain, M. (1976). *The Unabridged Mark Twain*. Running Press.

Chapter 6
Nursing an adult survivor of childhood sexual abuse

Fritha Irwin

This is a personal account of my experience of nursing Hannah, an adult survivor of childhood sexual abuse, during her thirteen-month treatment at the Cassel Hospital. We developed a very intense relationship which was, at times, extremely distressing for me. This distress was, however, balanced by warm, lighter moments and a feeling of progress with the patient.

Hannah taught me a great deal about how damaging childhood experiences can be upon the adult capacity to form relationships. Steele (1990: p. 26) suggests:

> Probably the most tragic sequel to sexual abuse is the pervasive, depressive feeling that one can never enter into a comfortable adult life and that rewarding, intimate relationships are impossible to achieve. Any attempt to be close with another person is perceived as dangerous.

I have been able to use this knowledge while nursing other adult survivors of childhood sexual abuse. Through sharing this learning with others, I hope they will be able to make use of it in their own work.

Hannah's story

Hannah was born in Devon and had two brothers. Her mother was a nurse and her father an electrician. When she was eight years old, her parents' marriage failed. Hannah and one brother stayed with their mother, while the other brother went to live with his father, stepmother and two stepbrothers. Hannah's mother had a history of mental health problems and became unable to care for her children. Hannah was soon abandoned by her mother. She vividly described how she had been left, one night, on her aunt's doorstep with a label attached to her coat.

This abandonment led to Hannah going to live with her father and stepfamily. She was then sexually abused by her two stepbrothers until the age of eighteen. It was then that she joined the army in order to get away from home. She had a successful army career and, at the age of 24, she married Charles, who was also in the army. Initially, their marriage was a success but their relationship deteriorated when they contemplated having a baby. It was at this point that Hannah's difficulties became apparent. She began to experience intense sleep disturbances and became anorexic and bulimic. She also began to abuse laxatives and alcohol. She and Charles started to have physical fights as well as horrific verbal arguments. They made a mutual decision to separate; Charles felt that they would destroy each other if they remained together. The couple were living in Germany at this time and Hannah decided to return to England in order to seek treatment for her problems.

On her return to England, Hannah had several courses of treatment in acute psychiatric settings. She had engaged in some outpatient psychotherapy but had become overwhelmed by the intense feelings stirred up by the treatment and this led to a serious suicide attempt. Her psychiatrist felt that she required a more contained setting in which her treatment could be safely pursued. He decided that an inpatient unit offering psychotherapy would be appropriate for her. She was thus referred to the Cassel Hospital.

Hannah's outpatient assessment and preadmission home visit

Treatment at the Cassel Hospital involves intensive psychosocial nursing, psychoanalytically oriented psychotherapy and participation in the therapeutic community. The assessment of a prospective patient is undertaken by both a psychotherapist and a senior psychosocial nurse. These assessments indicated that Hannah could gain from treatment at the Cassel Hospital and so arrangements were made for her admission.

It is believed to be important that patients should retain connections outside of the hospital while they are undergoing treatment. For this reason, it is a condition of treatment that patients have a home to return to at weekends. This condition supports the belief that patients are functioning adults who can manage some time away from the hospital. It also encourages them to face their difficulties at home and then bring these problems back to the hospital to work on with their nurses, psychotherapists and other patients, during the week.

Hannah's own home was still in Germany, so she arranged to stay on a temporary basis with friends, until she had obtained more permanent housing. It was to these friends' house that I went, accompanied by a current inpatient, to visit her before her admission to hospital. These visits are routine and provide prospective patients with the opportunity to meet two members of the therapeutic community and to hear something about the hospital life and its philosophy. They also offer the visitors a chance to learn a little about the prospective patient and then to inform the rest of the community of their difficulties before they arrive. This latter aspect is always made clear to the prospective patient during the visit.

When we visited Hannah, she was wary and unwelcoming. She made slightly more contact with the patient who was with me, but I was obviously viewed with great suspicion. I was left feeling very uncomfortable and could not understand why Hannah had taken such a dislike to me. I now think that Hannah saw me as an authority figure and, in view of the way previous authority figures in her life had let her down (her parents), it is perhaps not surprising that she felt unable to trust me.

Hannah was underweight, seemed younger than her age and had a boyish appearance. She had very short hair and was dressed in trousers and a baggy sweater. Through my experience of working with women who have been sexually abused as children, I have noticed how they often present an asexual appearance. Perhaps this is a way of denying their femininity and of repelling any sexual approach.

Hannah said very little about her problems during our visit and reacted angrily when I broached the subject of her diet and weight, denying any concerns. She alluded briefly to her difficulties in sleeping in response to the information that she would be sharing a room. She asked very few questions about the treatment or about the way of life in the Cassel Hospital.

Hannah's four-week inpatient assessment

Hannah was admitted to the hospital the following week for a four-week assessment period. This is an important part of treatment. The patients have time to decide whether they wish to continue with treatment after having experienced it for a month. The staff are given the opportunity to make an assessment about whether the hospital offers an appropriate form of treatment for them.

Hannah immediately made an impact upon the community by refusing to eat or drink, despite an expectation that everyone attends and eats meals. As she did not become dehydrated, it is very likely that she was drinking when out of the view of others. However, her behaviour generated a great deal of anxiety in me and a strong wish to 'look after her' by ensuring adequate nutrition and hydration. I think that Hannah's refusal to eat or drink was connected with her mother's inability to care for her and the resulting need in Hannah to generate caring in someone else (me) as compensation. She may have also been testing out whether I would care for her.

In her paper, 'Abuser and abused', Jane Milton (1994) describes the connection between eating disorders and a history of childhood sexual abuse. There is also a connection between an abused child's relationship with its mother and the development of eating disorders.

Hannah attended the other daily activities of the hospital, such as unit and community meetings and her individual therapy sessions. These meetings are an opportunity for patients to share their difficulties and feelings. However, Hannah was unable to participate verbally. She sat near the door, her head down and her legs swinging violently, thus silently communicating her fury at us and effectively keeping others at a distance. Other patients found her intimidating and unapproachable. If she was spoken to, Hannah seemed to perceive this as a verbal attack and stormed out of the room. This left us all feeling impotent in trying to understand and support her with her difficulties. I believe this feeling of impotence in me and in others was a reflection of Hannah's own experience whilst undergoing the abuse. She had been impotent to prevent it occurring.

Several times during the assessment period Hannah packed her bags in order to leave the hospital, but never actually did so. I think this behaviour was a reflection of her inner ambivalence about committing herself to what would be a long and painful treatment, as she began to face up to the awfulness of what had happened to her as a child.

My experience of working with Hannah during her assessment was difficult and bewildering. She was willing to spend time with me but gave me no eye contact. She was often silent and seemed furiously angry. I thought that her anger and hatred towards me was probably a reflection of her anger and hatred towards her parents who had not protected her from the abuse. Her perception of me did not seem based on reality and, therefore, may have been associated with her previous experience. Brendan McCarthy (1988: p. 113) suggests that: 'Incest victims frequently exhibit very strong and even overwhelming feelings of hate . . . it is usually prominent in the victim's attitude to professionals.'

Each attempted conversation with Hannah ended up with me feeling that I had done or said something awful to her. Hannah would frequently run away from me, swearing and, at times, overturning furniture as she left. My nursing work at this time was to establish a care plan in collaboration with Hannah, in order to help her to begin to address her difficulties. Among these were her low weight and appalling diet. When I tried to weigh Hannah in order to establish a healthy target weight for her to aim towards, her reaction was extreme. She refused to look at the scales or to let me read them properly. She rushed out of the room shouting and swearing and, subsequently, burst into tears. It was important for me to retain my sense of why this simple task of weighing her was so difficult – her self-starvation could have been life-threatening – and to recognize that what I wanted to do was caring and not abusive, which was how I then felt.

Another area of nursing work with Hannah was her disturbed nights. This was a problem which continued for many months into treatment. The disturbance was manifest as nightmares, which occurred every night. However, it seemed to me as if all the worry about this problem was mine, while Hannah was passive and uninvolved in thinking about how to change the situation. She presented herself as the victim of an awful event, rather than as an adult who wanted to confront the problem. The nightmares were extremely distressing to witness. Hannah shouted and screamed at people to 'go away' whilst thrashing around violently. She scratched at her face, leaving it covered in blood. She was very difficult to rouse. This usually took between 10 and 15 minutes, during which time those around her felt compelled to restrain her from further self-inflicted injury, as well as to offer comfort. The need for physical restraint was felt by those involved as if it were a repetition of Hannah's abuse during which she was also restrained. As Hannah vigorously rejected any physical contact during the day, one could speculate that this was her perverse adult way of obtaining and allowing physical contact.

Hannah's assessment meeting

Four weeks after Hannah's admission, the staff team held the assessment meeting. Her psychotherapist noted that Hannah had a long history of perverse and abusing relationships, which she was re-enacting within the treatment setting. She felt Hannah's needs were being projected on to those around her, causing great anxiety, while she herself remained unconcerned. Any suggestion of need within her was unbearable for her.

The staff group decided to offer Hannah treatment with the expectation that she would actively take on responsibilities within the community as a way of developing relationships with others. She was also expected to start talking to others about her difficulties and her feelings. The staff told Hannah that we felt it would be difficult for her to change and that during treatment there was a risk that she might feel suicidal. Hannah decided to accept treatment.

Nursing Hannah

As treatment progressed, Hannah slowly began to build relationships with others and reluctantly to allow them to support her. This was achieved through Hannah's involvement in the community life, by taking part, for example, in cooking with a supper team, and by being encouraged to join social activities.

My first indication that she was beginning to see me as I am, rather than as an abusing authority figure, was when she came to my defence one evening. I was being verbally and almost physically attacked by another patient. Hannah was able to see that this behaviour was totally inappropriate and told the other patient so. She also prevented the patient from making any physical contact with me. Once the situation had calmed down, I told Hannah that I had been touched by her support.

Hannah gradually began to show me her more vulnerable, caring side and slowly we progressed to being able to share a joke. I had the feeling that she was beginning to trust me and to believe that I could care about her. As a result, she became less hostile towards me and allowed me to get to know other aspects of her personality. She became more able to accept my nursing work as an indication that I did care about her, rather than as an attack upon her. Her eating difficulties and alcohol and laxative abuse slowly decreased, although the laxative misuse reoccurred during particularly difficult times in her treatment. Milton (1994) describes how survivors of sexual abuse often feel that there is something awful inside them and abuse laxatives as a way of ejecting this horror. Once Hannah was able to talk about the awful feelings inside her, she felt less compelled to use laxatives. A similar improvement occurred once she was able to take and hold on to something good from her relationships; she then began to eat properly and to stop vomiting, thus deriving more goodness from food.

Her passivity about her nightmares persisted for seven months. It is a reflection of how powerfully persuasive Hannah could be that the staff were drawn into a perverse agreement that she should have a room of her own for a while. This is completely contrary to the community's philosophy. Hannah refused to discuss her night disturbance during the day, even with her psychotherapist. I became increasingly frustrated with my inability to help her, as well as with her passivity. I knew, from past experience, that, if she was able to talk during the day, her nights would become more settled. I encouraged her roommates to tell her how distressing the nightmares were to observe, in the hope that some realization of the effect she was having on people who were important to her would motivate her into actively pursuing some resolution to the problem. It was important for Hannah to accept that the resolution of this problem rested within her. Eventually, she managed to discuss this issue with her psychotherapist, but it was very traumatic for her because the content of the nightmares appeared to be a re-enactment of her childhood sexual abuse. Gradually, her nights became more peaceful and settled. Without the support and challenges from patients and staff to face this issue, I believe that Hannah would have had many more months of awful distress at night.

One aspect of Hannah's treatment which I believe had an important impact upon our relationship was that her psychotherapist left the hospital during her stay. This meant that, for three months, Hannah had no individual psychotherapy sessions and she felt unable fully to utilize the group therapy sessions which were offered in their place. As a consequence, I was drawn into discussing areas with Hannah which would have been more appropriately talked about in therapy sessions.

With great pain, Hannah described to me some of the details of her sexual abuse. It had taken her many years to be able to talk about it, so I felt I had to listen to her and support her with those disclosures. However, I found it extremely distressing to hear the story and needed support from my colleagues in order to be able to deal with it. I felt great sadness for Hannah, and a rage towards those who had subjected her to such vile experiences. It was important for her that I believed her and that I was able to tolerate listening to her experience. I believe it was also important for her to know of my feelings in response to her story. As a result, she said that she felt I valued her as a person worth caring about. She was able to build upon this experience to share some of her story with other patients and to receive similar caring from them. This support from other community members was essential in allowing Hannah to face up to her past. Gradually, she was able to tolerate others seeing her distress and vulnerability and to learn that they would not take advantage of the situation. This had not been her experience when her vulnerability as a child had been a factor in the abuse recurring.

As a result of becoming involved in listening to Hannah's story I neglected, to a certain extent, my role as her psychosocial nurse, which should have focused on practical issues. By this stage of Hannah's treatment, I was encouraging her to establish a home for herself, to think about employment and to consider the option of marital therapy with Charles. He had remained in touch with Hannah whilst still living in Germany. This marital work would have involved meetings with staff, Charles and Hannah to discuss their relationship. Once I realized that I had become less active in my nursing work, I concentrated again on these practical tasks, working alongside Hannah. My role was to try to empower Hannah to make her own decisions and not to make them for her.

Work had always been important to Hannah because I think her work identity was the only one about which she felt sure. She easily found part-time work while still having treatment and went into full-time employment after her discharge.

Hannah became very active in finding accommodation for herself. This was a problem area because she had been out of England for several years. She explored all possibilities open to her, even writing to her local MP for his support in obtaining council housing. This had the desired result and she established a home for herself before leaving the hospital.

Charles and Hannah

The issue of family meetings with Charles was far more contentious. It was easy to forget that Hannah was married because she rarely mentioned Charles voluntarily. However, he was coming to England on leave and wanted to spend a week's holiday with her. She eventually decided that she would like a meeting to take place with her, Charles, her consultant psychotherapist and myself. Hannah was extremely anxious before this meeting but both she and Charles were able to talk openly. It became clear that Hannah had only allowed Charles to become emotionally close to her for a short time and had then pushed him away, leaving him feeling rejected and angry. As they had never really discussed Hannah's past, it was hard for Charles to understand her behaviour. He had some knowledge about the sexual abuse but she had never told him the full story. They decided they would have their week away and try to enjoy just being together.

We all met again on their return from holiday. They had each experienced the time away quite differently. Charles had enjoyed it on the whole but Hannah had found it extremely difficult to enjoy herself and to be constantly with her husband. It was hard for them to listen to each other and to respect the other's point of view. The issue of their future together remained undecided. Charles was due to return to England and he wanted to try to re-establish their marriage. The relationship was an area which would require further work once Hannah was discharged from treatment. It is important to note that Hannah's difficulties had originally become apparent when she and Charles had considered starting a family of their own. The thought of children must have stirred up very painful memories of her own experiences as a child, which she was unable to cope with at that time.

Approaching discharge

Hannah's last few weeks of treatment were hard for her. She felt rejected and abandoned by the staff. Her response to these feelings was to retreat into the angry, attacking Hannah we had known on admission. Her previous experience of being abandoned as a child meant that she found it very difficult to deal with separations.

However, she was also able to reflect upon her experience within the therapeutic community and to recognize how much she had gained. I felt that it was the right time for her to leave the hospital. I had grown very fond of her and was sad to say goodbye. I also felt that she had gained enough knowledge of her perverse ways of relating to have the opportunity of a more fulfilling life. She was now aware that she did not have to be a passive victim of others but could take control of her own life. She had also learnt to talk about her own needs and had developed real intimate relationships. These positive skills would be taken with her into her life outside the hospital.

What did I learn from Hannah?

Primarily, I learned how difficult it is to work with a patient who has had past experiences similar to Hannah. It takes patience, a conviction that one is doing the right thing, and time to establish a relationship.

I have already mentioned how the hate and anger felt by sexually abused people towards their abusers is often directed towards those who try to help them. This can be very difficult to withstand at times.

Milton (1994: p. 243) describes how 'The patient is at times in her current life the abuser, and then at times the abused'. This certainly explains why I often felt as if I were abusing Hannah.

Jehu (1994) discusses some consequences of childhood sexual abuse which lead to the patient either being passive and submissive or compensating by being overcontrolling. These traits, too, can make these patients very difficult to work with, and must be faced in order to develop mutual relationships.

McCarthy (1988) stresses the importance of a dependable structure within the treatment programme of patients who have been sexually abused. I, therefore, had to be constant and dependable when nursing Hannah. At times, when she was angry with me, this was difficult to maintain because I did not want to be with her.

Powerful feelings about being rejected were stirred up in Hannah whenever I or her psychotherapist went on annual leave. She experienced the holiday as a re-enactment of her mother's abandonment of her. The anticipation of absences is, therefore, vital when working with patients who have had similar experiences.

Several physical symptoms common to adult survivors of sexual abuse were exhibited by Hannah. These included eating disorders, laxative and alcohol abuse, and self-injury (at night, during her nightmares). It was important for me to express my concern to Hannah about these destructive behaviours. Through this verbal feedback, she began to realize the effect of her behaviour on other people. As she began to develop some self-esteem, she also began to realize how damaging she was being to herself.

Finally, I also learned that, if one is able to persist, nursing an adult survivor of childhood sexual abuse can be a most rewarding experience.

My support

Nursing Hannah was often personally distressing and so my support systems were vital in enabling me to continue in my work with her. Regular weekly supervision with the senior nurse on the unit helped me to understand the dynamics within my relationship with Hannah; for example, why I was made to feel I was abusing her when I was simply trying to care for her. Once I understood the dynamics, they became easier to tolerate.

Regular communication with other staff, particularly Hannah's psychotherapist, was also important. This was achieved via staff meetings and review meetings of Hannah's treatment. It meant that the anxiety that Hannah projected into me was shared by discussion with other staff; this made it more bearable for me when her behaviour in the community became more disturbed. At such times, she was usually discussing very difficult issues in her therapy sessions. Communication with her therapist made me aware of this connection and I was then more able to support Hannah.

It was also vital for me to express my feelings to Hannah. When I felt impotent or angry, these were usually her feelings projected into me. She had to learn to recognize these feelings as her own and accept them herself.

I was also supported by other patients in the community when I had to confront Hannah about her behaviour. This made a difficult situation more manageable.

My nursing colleagues supported me, validating my work at times when I doubted it, and mopping up my tears when necessary! This support was both formal and informal.

I hope this account of my experience of nursing Hannah shows how we were able to face difficult issues together and to survive the distress. Ultimately, any credit for this must go to Hannah. It was she who took the risk to involve herself in treatment, knowing that it would be very painful and not knowing what the outcome would be.

References

Jehu, D. (1994). *Patients as Victims. Sexual Abuse in Psychotherapy and Counselling.* John Wiley.
McCarthy, B. (1988). Are incest victims hated? *Psychoanal. Psychother.*, 3, 113–120.

Milton, J. (1994). Abuser and abused: perverse solutions following childhood abuse. *Psychoanal. Psychother.*, 8, 243–255.

Steele, B.F. (1990). The sexual maltreatment of children. In *Adult Analysis and Childhood Sexual Abuse* (H.B. Levine, ed.), Analytic Press.

Chapter 7
The use of self in child protection work

Vicki Mills

The following chapter attempts to explore how psychosocial understanding can be used in conjunction with current child care legislation
and practice guidelines. It explores the effect of statutory obligations on
the relationship between the social worker and the client. It concludes
that it is the use of self that is the most important therapeutic tool and
highlights some of the problems for practitioners in the field of child
protection.

For a child protection practitioner, the casework dilemma is to maintain a balance between statutory obligation and therapeutic value, while
remaining child-focused. There are a number of factors to be considered
which can seem to be in contrast and competition with one another. It can
be difficult to ascertain facts about abuse, which may lead to a criminal
prosecution, while at the same time trying to establish a working relationship with a family. However, it is part of a thorough investigation to
establish what abuse, if any, has taken place.

A working definition of abuse might be that the basic needs of the child
are not being met through avoidable acts of either commission or
omission. This is based on accepting that a child has a basic need for
physical care and protection, physical and emotional growth, love and
security, intellectual development and stimulation. If, after a full investigation, a multidisciplinary child protection case conference decides to
place a child's name on the Child Protection Register, the child can only
be registered as suffering or likely to suffer one or a combination of the
following categories of abuse: physical, emotional, sexual, or neglect.

The purpose of the Register is to ensure that regular multi-agency conferences are held about the child and plans made to protect the child, while alerting other agencies that a particular child is vulnerable. Most children who are placed on the Register are not removed from home. Others are removed for short periods while initial investigations are made.

Child care legislation and policy guidelines

Child care legislation was overhauled and mostly rewritten into the 1989 Children Act. The Act clearly defines local authorities' responsibilities towards children and families. For example, Section 47 of the Act describes local authorities' duty to investigate when there are child protection concerns. The Act also advises what should be done to safeguard or promote a child's welfare, including making an application to a family court for a child to be removed from home. When the plan is permanently to remove a child, adoption is the preferred option, sometimes with parental contact. However, this decision-making process is lengthy, with many legal stages and court appearances.

In addition to the 1989 Children Act, other legislation was introduced in the 1980s which affects social work practice peripherally, such as: the Police and Criminal Evidence Act 1984; the Access to Personal Files Act 1987; and the Prohibition of Female Circumcision Act 1985, to name just a few. Following the Children Act, the Department of Health, the Social Services Inspectorate and individual local authorities have issued a myriad of policy and procedure documents regarding standards and good practice in child protection work, such as equal opportunity guidelines, because many of the families involved with social services belong to ethnic or other minority groups. Most local authorities have developed policies to ensure that permanence is considered in plans for a child's future and that these plans should not 'drift', either by default or by an unrealistically optimistic assessment of the parents' ability to provide 'good enough' parenting. The notion of 'good enough' parenting, which has been explored by Winnicott (1964) and Bettleheim (1987), describes parenting that is sufficient to allow a child to develop and flourish, both physically and emotionally. A permanent decision should be made as soon as the parents' parenting ability has been assessed and rehabilitation considered or tried.

Self-protective systems

The procedural context listed above can seem stifling and bureaucratic when the worker is actually dealing with the client. It can be difficult to remain focused on the child at risk when the fear of failing in the procedure can take precedence. The fear of public and professional reprisal if you 'get it wrong' is justified when consideration is given to the public enquiries that have followed the deaths of children. Many have been critical of individual professionals for not following the correct procedure and failing to protect a child. Without the assistance of sophisticated supervision and training, child protection practitioners can hide behind this system, albeit unconsciously, to protect themselves from the discomfort and distress of the abuse and the abuser. The bureaucracy and the procedures involved can be so time-consuming that the focus shifts from the child to the system, and the fear of failing becomes the motivating factor in the work. This, in turn, allows workers to distance themselves from the feelings of anger and disgust towards the perpetrator of the abuse and thus helps them, even if based on false premise, to develop relationships with the perpetrator. When this happens and it is not picked up in supervision, a system of collusion develops and the abuse becomes minimized. This, in turn, prevents an abuser from feeling responsible for his or her actions, and the child cannot be protected effectively from a danger that is not recognized and not seen to exist.

In this context, it is understandable why the dynamic process is often ignored, as is the effect of the worker's feeling, about his or her own sense of childhood and experiences of being parented. If these emotions are explored, considerable discomfort, such as painful childhood memories, can be experienced by the worker. These may not be containable within a system that is fraught and busy and has the real task to complete of carrying out numerous child protection investigations.

Psychosocial nursing at the Cassel Hospital differs by ensuring that time is taken to acknowledge and understand these important emotions and to encourage the nursing staff to understand the effects that their work has upon them. This, in turn, may persuade nurses to seek psychotherapeutic help in their own right to cope with the personal issues that the work can evoke. A social services department is culturally different and, predictably, has a high turnover of staff and a high sickness record, which may indicate high levels of unresolved stress and anxiety.

Psychodynamic practice is no longer encouraged in most social work settings. The last course teaching social work theory in this way was discontinued in 1994. Training now centres mostly on case management and the expectation is that social workers will 'buy in' the services a client may need (for example, counselling) from other agencies, often in the voluntary sector. This further separates the local authority social worker from developing in-depth relationships with clients.

Menzies (1960) identified this self-protective process as it related to student nurses in general training, but there are comparisons in social work. Menzies writes of the resurgence in the nurse of infantile phantasies that are opposing in nature, the libidinal and the aggressive, the latter being death-dealing and destructive. There are aspects of child protection that are repugnant and lead to feelings of aggression in the practitioner and, at times, disgust for the alleged abuser. Invariably, this is dealt with indirectly by splitting clients into the bad or the sick, and, in this way, the practitioner can remain healthy and good. As the power for decision making about the child lies with the professionals, the alleged abuser can become further paralysed and the healthy, good and nurturing aspects ignored. These aspects are seen only to belong to the professionals. This system can suit abusing clients and practitioners alike because it allows the former to disown their actions, and project feelings of guilt and depression, anxiety, fear and disgust of the abuse on to the practitioner. Within this dynamic, there can be little sharing of management or decision making about the child between parent(s) and social worker. Klein (1946) describes these adult defensive mechanisms, and their origins in the psychological development of children, in the way they deal with anger and anxiety.

The Children Act 1989 and the guidelines that followed (Department of Health, 1991), have gone some way in establishing firm principles to ensure that social workers must work in partnership with families and that compulsory action can only be taken when voluntary agreements cannot be made. However, by and large, such documents set the standard with little regard to the dynamic process created, or to the defence mechanisms used by client or practitioner.

Responsibility within child protection is the constant hot potato which individuals are eager to pass on wherever possible. Although accountability within the various multidisciplinary agencies is generally well defined, a vague sense of distrust or criticism often pervades within and between the different agencies. Menzies (1960) describes this well:

> Complaints about irresponsibility stem from a collusive system of denial, splitting and projecting, that is culturally acceptable to, and indeed culturally required . . . Irresponsible impulses that cannot be controlled are attributed to juniors . . . painfully severe attitudes to these impulses and a burdensome sense of responsibility are attributed to seniors.

There are parallels in the way that responsibility and culpability are dealt with between professional and client. Each, on one level, is trying to persuade the other to 'own' and deal with the abusive behaviour. When this cannot be resolved within the casework, the ultimate decisions about children are made collectively by the statutory agencies, with the courts acting as the final sanction.

Working towards change

The process by which a social worker reaches a decision about what recommendation to make after a child protection investigation is by undertaking a 'comprehensive assessment'. The Department of Health guidelines (1988) for social workers completing such an assessment proposes a very thorough selection of questions such as questions about family background and attitude towards the child(ren) during pregnancy. The guidelines suggest formats and the use of genograms to establish visually where a client belongs within the family. This procedure is followed, with small variations to suit different circumstances, and it is an efficient tool in the collection of necessary information. In my own experience, this way of investigating acts is a necessary short cut because it crosses all the boundaries of 'usual' social interaction. By asking direct and personal questions, the social worker can collect much information about a family and how its members function and interact.

In therapeutic work, the therapist allows the client to set the pace and to reveal secrets and truths, or not, depending on how much risk the client is prepared to take. In a comprehensive assessment, as part of a child protection investigation, the reverse is true. The social worker's questions about highly personal matters have a dramatic effect on the relationship with the client. Often clients will have had poor or abusive parenting as children and will have been left with a negative view of their parents and will carry this memory deep within. In reality, the experiences of being parented may or may not have been bad, but he or she feels that the experience was negative and, therefore, carries a bad parent within. In this context, the 'bad' parent is a psychological construct that can include both actual and imagined parental deficits. The assessment process can stir up these feelings and memories. The client will have little choice about taking part in the assessment and the skill for the social worker lies in containing the powerful emotions raised.

Winnicott (1964) describes the role of containment as a hold and support unit by which one person flourishes and, in turn, can nurture because of the support of another, such as a mother who can care for a baby because of support from the father or from her family. Weddell (1968) describes the role of the Cassel nurse who 'hold/supports' the mothers he or she works with, so that they, in turn, can care for their children. This is an essential part of nursing at the Cassel Hospital and the technique transfers well to social work with families. The social worker will need to empower the client to make full use of the most mature functioning part of the personality and, in turn, try not to see the client as all 'bad'. Nurses at the Cassel Hospital constantly encourage patients to use their strengths and capabilities to overcome depressed and destructive feelings. In child protection work, the same encouragement and support are essential when working with abusive or neglectful parents, to ensure that their parenting becomes safer.

There needs to be a point at which there is some mutual exchange and some recognition of each others' vulnerability and humanity, while maintaining a professional relationship. Social workers also need to be very clear about their own sense of internalized parents and childhood, and not to be searching for a vicarious resolution to their own childhood traumas. As child abuse is an assault on our own internalised child, work in this field can sometimes seem to be appealing to those with unresolved conflicts. In my experience, the assessment process falls short when this is not recognized, where supervision and training are inadequate and when clients cannot be contained. At times, it is impossible for a particular worker to contain clients. Sometimes, the parents are too psychologically fragmented to engage in the assessment process; for example, they may become violent or are recognized to have serious mental health problems.

This containment is pivotal if any change is to be attained. Alternating feelings of goodness and badness will be projected towards the social worker, who will need to understand, rather than merely react, to such emotions. In A *Fragment on Mothering* Tom Main (1968) suggests that mothers are often perceived as either Madonnas (pure, loving, asexual, nurturing) or witches (hateful, destructive and promiscuous). In my experience, every effort will be made by the client to view both the social worker and the role of parent in this way. The social worker may be seen as the idealized Madonna or the wicked witch. The client may attempt to avoid any effort by the professionals to scrutinize his or her parenting. This maintains the split between good and bad, and the client can disown and project negative acts and emotions and protect him or herself from the pain of dealing with the abuse. Similarly, the social worker needs to be wary of falling into the role of 'good', uncritical parent, and of colluding with the client to ignore the abuse, or of being unrealistic about the client's parenting ability. Equally, the social worker should not become the 'bad' overcritical parent and reawaken earlier experiences in the client that stem from memories of being parented, unless time can be spent on understanding or working through the subsequent effects. This, of course, moves the focus away from the child and on to the parent, and is not part of a protection investigation.

The changes that families make when children are deemed to be at risk seem to fall into two categories and can happen over a number of years. First, parents who can face their own internal parent and exorcise their own trauma develop far greater empathy and better parenting skills. This is obviously the hope of any therapeutic work because the effect of the change becomes fully integrated into the client's personality. In reality, this is less often achieved when working with abusing families, for many reasons, but mostly, I believe, because their own experiences have been too traumatic. The shift away from using psychodynamic principles in the training of social workers and a reduction in social work posts with a resultant increase in workload, have also taken their toll.

For some families who cannot change, the child may be permanently removed. There are situations when children are returned or remain in unsafe or abusive situations because the parent(s) cannot be engaged and the abuse or neglect cannot be proved, or because the emotional attachment is so great that to separate the child would be adding to the abuse. This is often the case for an older child. In large sibling groups, the local authority can rarely offer a good enough alternative to home in the immediate future. For example, it may not be able to keep siblings together because there is no available placement. This situation is more common since the 1989 Children Act was introduced, because the Act states that the wishes of the young person must be taken into account. The Act further places responsibility on the local authority to prove that what it can offer is a better alternative. This is called the 'assumption of no order', which means that no order will be granted by a court unless it can be seen to offer a better and preferred option for the children.

A less fundamental change, a change in behaviour, can be acquired, which improves parenting ability to a safer level; this may enable the child to remain within the natural family. The reasons why this might be achieved are many, but they include education, such as teaching basic child-care skills, and offering practical support such as welfare rights assistance. However, continuing to work with families over long periods and containing them seem to be the main components behind such change. The determinants for the abuse remain, in part at least, but the response is different. By not reacting thoughtlessly to the attempts to project, to split, to deny, and to alienate and disgust, the social worker helps the client to behave differently. Maturity, confidence and self-esteem can improve by helping the abuser to 'own' destructive impulses and anger. In short, the social worker can offer another kind of parenting to the client to enable him or her to develop a safer environment for the children. The parent's internalized 'bad' parent may remain, but he or she has some experience that another kind of parenting is possible. My work, or rather my failings, with Mona and her children illustrate this. Mona's name has been changed to protect her identity.

Mona: a case study

I worked with Mona and her children for five years and experienced an emotional roller coaster along the way, due to Mona's great 'neediness' and an uncanny ability she seemed to have in making great demands upon me when I was least able to respond (for example, when I was dealing with a crisis concerning another client).

Mona is in her early thirties and has four daughters; two of whom were born while I was working with her. She is a single parent living on benefit and is of West Indian and Asian parentage.

Mona's childhood was violent; her parents fought and she was often caught in the crossfire. Her father sexually abused her and her mother neglected her, physically and emotionally. Mona has three sisters who are all happily settled with families and offer her a lot of support and help in caring for her children. Mona has little contact with her parents and her father is currently serving a life sentence for murder. As a child, Mona feels that she was treated less favourably than her sisters, and, in adult life, she has become the person in the family who seems to take on the negative aspects for all of them. Mona, it would seem, is the family's emotional sacrifice and scapegoat who enables the mother and sisters to function fairly well.

Mona was raped when she was aged 18 and her eldest child was the outcome of this assault. She married at 20 and her second child was born two years later. The marriage ended after four years of domestic violence and Mona became involved with the father of her youngest two daughters. He has mild learning disabilities. He beat her regularly, and this necessitated several house moves to different secret addresses, in order to separate her from him.

Mona has regular episodes of severe depression that have required hospitalization. During these times, she has been violent to the girls and emotionally abusive and neglectful. When she is well, she provides a standard of care that is just good enough. Without the help and support of their aunts, the girls would have needed to be removed from their mother's care.

Over the five years during which I worked with the family, Mona received several beatings from her partner, which always presented as crises and were followed by periods of depression. Mona would arrive at my office with the expectation that I would help her to recover, deal with her distress and the fears of her daughters, help her to deal with the police and decisions around prosecution, and help her to effect the support of her sisters. She could not ask them directly for help because her envy of them was too great, but she knew that, if I was worried for the children, I would call the extended family together. In effect, Mona gave up and was unable to react to the world unless she provoked a crisis. She almost failed to get to hospital to give birth to her fourth child, but waited until she was in the advanced stage of labour. She called me, and together we made it to the hospital with only minutes to spare.

During the periods of depression Mona could be dangerous and unpredictable. She talked about 'pressure in my head' and needing 'to flip' to describe the rage within her that could erupt into violence. She would appear to lose control and any inhibitions. One day she tried to strangle her 10-year old and, although the attack was not life-threatening, it was terrifying. Another time, she tried to smash and jump through the window of my office on the second floor. When Mona was depressed, she neglected her children. She would not feed them and sent them to their rooms far too early at night, so that she did not have to have contact with them. During these periods, Mona and the children demanded an excessive amount of my time.

Throughout the first four years, the family and I contained the distress and the crises. We worked closely to ensure that the girls were safe and to help Mona to make full use of the healthy aspects of her personality, such as her organizational ability and her love for the girls. Mona's sisters and I organized an elaborate system of 'shared care' for the children when their mother was unable to cope. If they were worried, the older children would sometimes initiate our involvement and knew how to contact me and their aunts, with whom they would go and stay for lengthy periods. Sometimes, Mona went too. I had wanted to put this arrangement on a more formal basis via the family proceedings court but, under the 'assumption of no order', I would have failed to obtain an order. No one in the family, including the children, wanted one and I would not have been able to provide a better alternative with an order than without one.

By the end of the fourth year, Mona and the children were more settled and had moved to a very nice property in a new area. Mona's violent partner had no idea where they were. All the children were settled in school or nursery care, leaving Mona more time to relax. For the first time, it was possible to look at helping Mona to take control of events and not to be a victim of circumstance, which is how she felt. For Mona, it was impossible to accept her part in the events around her life and, given her childhood experiences of sexual abuse and neglect, there was a great deal of justification in her feeling this way. However, as the practical tasks of moving house and becoming more settled were completed, Mona became increasingly distressed and depressed and, as a consequence, abusive towards the children. It is impossible to know why Mona became more depressed at this time. Her circumstances were more settled and she seemed to find this unnerving. I believe it was because she had time to think and was not merely responding to crises. The danger of domestic violence had disappeared and Mona had to own her destructive impulses and could no longer project these on to her partner. For the first time she had an opportunity to change her role of being a victim.

My response to this was, frankly, one of irritation. I felt I had moved mountains to make things better and had contained and supported her for long enough. A new counselling project for black women who had been victims of domestic violence was set up in the area at about this time and I decided to ask Mona if she would like me to refer her. She agreed, the referral was made, and I met the counsellor to define our respective roles. I would remain the primary worker for the children, but Mona would receive her support from the counselling project. My feelings of irritation turned to a feeling of relief and I chose to ignore my anger and annoyance that Mona was still being very demanding. I rationalized that it was 'sensible' for Mona to be referred to another professional. I felt that she had not made good use of my efforts to help her and wanted more from me. I failed to understand and to be sensitive to Mona's possible feelings of rejection. I failed to be perceptive about what my own feelings meant and merely responded to them. I used the 'system' and the culture in which I worked to justify this as the best use of my time and resources, and forgot how important it had been that I had 'carried' and 'contained' Mona for so long, and that we had an established relationship that had a therapeutic value in itself.

In retrospect, the outcome was predictable. Within two weeks, the new counsellor became the good, nurturing Madonna, the only person capable of understanding Mona and her predicament. I became the wicked witch who wanted to snatch away the children and who had never been of any value or help. Although I was intellectually aware that this was not so, my emotional response was to feel hurt and unappreciated. I had felt guilty about the relief I experienced in handing Mona over, and now I had a need to be punished, which Mona was fulfilling.

The new counsellor was inexperienced and was flattered by Mona's dramatic improvement in mood and unknowingly colluded with the split. Between them, they made a formal complaint about the service Mona had received from social services, which necessitated a case review by senior managers. After the initial period when Mona responded positively, her depression re-emerged. The counsellor became more and more anxious and admitted to feeling very frightened of Mona and her destructive depression, which she had previously denied. The result was chaotic, with the professionals in disagreement and all parties wishing to lay blame at each other's feet. When I used time in supervision, to consider privately some of the psychodynamic principles I have discussed, it was possible to make sense of what had happened. I had not taken the time to understand what my feelings meant nor had I realized how depleted my work with Mona had left me. It was possible to share some of this with Mona, as we met several times to talk and to repair our relationship.

Discussion and conclusion

For most of the time that I had known Mona, she had tried to establish an exclusive relationship with me at the expense of the girls, who were my primary clients. Her need for the containment and mothering that she had never received from her own mother was such that she transferred this on to me. I, as her own mother before, frustrated her by not being able to meet her needs, and her dependence upon me irritated me. I had failed to deal with this adequately and so her expectation of me as the all-encompassing, giving, maternal figure continued. When I failed her, I quickly became the wicked witch. I felt judgemental about her neglect of her daughters and allowed myself to take some responsibility away from Mona for the abuse by owning these critical feelings, and not examining them with her. I also reawakened Mona's critical parent within, to whom she had never felt truly acceptable or good enough. Mona was envious of my seemingly warm attitude and of my relationship with her daughters. I felt it necessary to question whether I was envious of her motherhood, as it was at this time that my own infertility became apparent. Working with abusing mothers became more difficult while I came to terms with this.

Mona experienced my referral to another person as a rejection. This further evoked childhood memories for her of feeling unacceptable and that no one could tolerate her destructiveness. In truth, I could not tolerate her destructive depression and felt that I had given her enough, and that she should be better after all my efforts. Rather than deal with this and question whether Mona had the capacity to get better, or whether I had a need always to succeed, I chose to rationalize my decision to refer Mona to another professional.

Mona has now moved to another borough permanently and therefore has another social worker, although much greater care was taken about handing the case over. Her children remain on the Child Protection Register, although I understand her parenting is not so worrying. She remains apart from her violent ex-partner and has not replaced him with another, violent or otherwise. This is an improvement for Mona, who has never remained outside a violent relationship for so long, almost five years. She still suffers from depression but is more stable. Her eldest daughter is now 16 years old and, predictably, is experiencing a difficult adolescence.

Without the theoretical grounding in psychotherapeutic principles, I would have found it impossible to work with Mona or others like her. If I could not understand behaviour by linking it to a client's past and childhood experience, and to the self-protective mechanisms employed, I would be mystified and unable to assess whether a child was at risk or not. Most of my clients do not refer themselves and can be angry about my intervention. If I could not understand their response as it relates to their earliest relationships, I could not engage with them without forming overly friendly and collusive relationships. This would avoid the primary task of assessing risk. Mostly, I cannot share this understanding with clients, as my job is not to interpret, but it provides me with the confidence to work with families who are dysfunctional.

I began to acquire this knowledge base at the Cassel Hospital, but this is only part of what the hospital taught me. Most importantly, it taught me about containing distress and that I need to experience and understand my own feelings and responses about work, however painful. As a general trained nurse, I was used to seeing patients as sick, incapable and infantilized. Work at the Cassel Hospital demonstrated that a person's symptom or sickness is only one aspect of that individual, who may have strengths and abilities and capacity for change that need to be nurtured and encouraged. I believe it is possible to develop relationships to facilitate this. Without this more optimistic view, working in child protection would be merely a form of social policing.

References

Bettleheim, B. (1987). *A Good Enough Parent*. Thames and Hudson.

Department of Health. (1988). *Protecting Children – a Guide for Social Workers Undertaking a Comprehensive Assessment*. HMSO.

Department of Health. (1991). *Working Together Under the Children Act 1989*. HMSO.

Klein, M. (1946). *Notes on some Schizoid Mechanisms*. In (1975). *Envy and Gratitude and other works 1946–1963* (pp. 1–24), Hogarth Press.

Klein, M. (1959). *Our Adult World and its Roots in Infancy*. In (1975). *Envy and Gratitude and Other Works 1946–1963* (M. Masud and R. Khan, eds.) (pp. 248–263), Hogarth Press.

Main, T. (1968). A Fragment on mothering. In *Psychosocial Nursing: Studies from the Cassel Hospital* (E. Barnes, ed.) pp. 143–155, Tavistock Publications.

Menzies, I.E.P. (1960). A case study in the functioning of social systems as a defence against anxiety: a study of the nursing service of a general hospital. *Hum. Relations*, **13**, 95–121.

Weddell, D. (1968). Family Centred Nursing. In *Psychosocial Nursing: Studies from the Cassel Hospital* (E. Barnes, ed.) pp. 137–142, Tavistock Publications.

Winnicott, D.W. (1964). *The Child, the Family and the Outside World*. Pelican.

Chapter 8
Mary's story

Ann Simpson

This chapter is an example of specialist nursing, developed on the Cassel nursing model, at the North Essex Child and Family Consultation Service. The core nursing function was working with families in the 'here and now' setting of their own homes, where a child's behaviour and difficulties in family relationships could be observed and interpreted within the context of daily family life. Active participation with families is particularly useful when parents and children are unable to put feelings into words. The focus of an activity can provide a platform for tensions to emerge. In order to do this work, health-care professionals require a knowledge of human emotional development, coupled with an understanding of psycho-dynamic processes, so that they can face the painful feelings and nurse fragile relationships gradually back to health.

Mary's story illustrates some of the principles of a psychosocial nursing model. The story is about supporting a woman to find her own strengths as a wife and mother, and to survive a life-threatening illness. It was important to have a framework, and yet also to be flexible. Mary and her family gained a sense of autonomy, which I think could be attributed to this model of nursing, in which the nurse–patient relationship is a focus, the healthy aspects of patients are encouraged, and the nurse attempts to work alongside the patient.

Colin is referred

When I first met Mary and Derek, their five-year-old son, Colin, had been referred to our service by the local social services department. Colin had an older brother, Jason, then aged six years and two younger sisters, Nancy, then aged three, and Stephanie, 18 months old. A social worker had been involved with the family since 1991 after a case conference was called because Colin had a black eye as a result of being hit by his father. The outcome of the conference was not to place Colin and the other children on the Child Protection Register; nevertheless, there was great concern about the physical and emotional welfare of all the children.

Colin was singled out by his parents as being the problem in the family. They felt the older brother, Jason, had never been a problem. The parents saw Nancy's apparent challenging behaviour at home as copying brother Colin. Stephanie, the baby, was not seen as having any difficulties, but the health visitor and community paediatrician had identified gross delay in her motor development, possibly due to the low level of stimulation in the household, and a reluctance of her parents to allow her to explore her environment. Stephanie at that time was grossly overweight and suffered from asthma.

Mary was in poor physical health; she was almost permanently tired, had kidney and asthmatic problems and was suffering recurrent out-breaks of boils and sores on her face and in her mouth.

The professionals involved thought that the family appeared to scapegoat Colin, and to see him as the cause of all the current parenting difficulties. Mary and Derek were questioning Colin's mental health state, saying he was 'mad', a 'nutter' and a 'schizophrenic'. All four children were understimulated at home. Their mother was very tired, and their father was a strict disciplinarian, particularly with Colin. There was both physical and verbal violence between Mary and Derek, which appeared to have a marked effect on the children. Mary was anxious about Derek's behaviour with the children, particularly in her absence, or when she was asleep in the early hours of the morning.

All the professionals involved (social worker, health visitor, general practitioner, community paediatrician, school teacher and nursery teacher) were very concerned that the basic needs of the children were not being met, and they feared also that Colin would be completely rejected by the family. These professionals put considerable work into the family over the next few months, with little or no effect. The referral letter to our service came, it seemed, as a last resort, with the referrer indicating the extreme pessimism felt by those involved. Colin was withdrawn and appeared depressed. Everything had been tried, to no avail. The referral and communication from the professionals involved with the family seemed to describe vividly something of the quality of the family relationships, the ways in which each family member tried to communicate, and the amount of deprivation the children were experiencing with parents unable to attend to their physical and emotional needs.

It seemed that the problems of the family were being pushed on to one member, a little five-year-old, whose only way of surviving and 'feeling alive', perhaps, was to urinate in drawers in his bedroom, defecate in the corner of his bedroom, hit and bully his younger sisters and be defiant of his parents. Behaviour like this will sometimes be the healthiest way of 'going on being' that a child can find in an otherwise inadequate emotional environment. Antisocial acts such as bedwetting and stealing indicate that, at any rate, momentarily there can be hope – hope of rediscovering a good enough internalized parent (Winnicott, 1964). Scapegoating one family member can, sometimes, be seen as the only way of holding things together until something is sorted out and, therefore, can have a positive as well as a negative effect.

If we look at problems of behaviour in children generally, it is likely that the behaviour has a specific emotional meaning. It may be an expression of deprivation, or show that frightening and aggressive feelings are not being contained.

With all families who are causing concern, we look not only at the interpersonal dynamics within the referred family, but also try to understand how these may be reflected among the professionals associated with the family. These dynamics, which are often unconscious, may either reflect the needs of the professionals or be a manifestation of the dynamic difficulties within the family. This is one way of understanding such situations, but, of course, it is not the only way.

Initial interview

When Colin was referred to our service, it was thought that I would be the most appropriate professional to make an initial assessment of the family. We thought I should meet the health visitor and social worker to hear from them directly about the work they had already tried to do with the family. The health visitor attended the meeting, but the social worker did not.

When I enquired about this later, the social worker told me she had forgotten. I therefore arranged another meeting with her, and Mary and Derek. This was to be a joint assessment about the difficulties Colin was presenting, and to decide whether our service could be of help. They all duly arrived for the appointment, but the social worker said she would have to leave after five minutes for a child protection visit. I wondered whether her absence reflected her sense of failure and a wish to rid herself of this family. Whatever the reason, I felt angry that she left me 'holding the baby'. In a sense, Mary, Derek and I were perhaps all experiencing 'being left to get on with it', and were, therefore, starting off from a similar position.

At this initial interview, it emerged that Mary had suffered severe postnatal depression after Colin's birth, and, for the first three months, Derek had seen to most of his care. Now, it seemed that Mary did all the talking, and Derek ignored any questions I asked of him. They both seemed invested in the idea that Colin, who was about to start school, was mentally ill.

I agreed with Mary and Derek to make an extended assessment. I would visit Mary and Colin and the two younger girls at home four times over the next consecutive weeks. Each visit was to be about an hour and 15 minutes, with planned appointment times.

Assessment visits

I found the visits difficult and, at times, overwhelming. I noted the very poor and dirty conditions of the home; the number of broken toys and furniture, the amount of distress expressed by Nancy and Stephanie, who were constantly crying and clinging to their mother. She, on one occasion, handled them very severely in my presence. Colin seemed very withdrawn. He would hide behind the settee, emerging from time to time to tear up books or hit his younger sisters.

I discovered that Mary drank a lot, which was something no one had told me about. She was in a desperately poor physical condition, had frequent headaches, boils on her face, and constant mouth ulcers. The children's physical hygiene was poor, and there was not enough money or food. I wondered where to begin. To single Colin out for specific help would only reinforce the idea that he was the family problem, and the most basic needs of the children would still not be met. After discussions with colleagues, I decided to work with Mary. If she could engage with me and feel supported by me, this might help her to look after the children. There was no doubt that she was the pivot around which the whole family revolved, and she was tired, ill and unable to eat properly.

One afternoon, Mary was drinking alcohol when I visited, and the children were so fractious that I was very anxious indeed about their care. I consulted one of my social worker colleagues on the team, and we decided together not to telephone the child protection team at our local social services department. I would write a letter to Mary that day (they were not on the telephone) expressing my concern about her and the current situation, and bringing forward my planned appointment for the following week from Thursday to Monday, hoping that this intervention would 'hold' things by showing Mary that she was very much on my mind. By the time I visited two days later, Mary was much less distressed and was much calmer with the children. This response to my intervention demonstrated that Mary could probably use the particular kind of nursing that I was offering.

Mary agreed to start meeting weekly with me, although it was ridiculed by Derek, and we embarked on a period of transformation in her and in the family's functioning.

After the assessment, Mary and I planned regular appointments at the clinic. This was so that she could have time, away from home, to explore the difficulties in the family. The girls could be looked after by a neighbour, and the clinic was a short walk from her home. She needed to value this time for herself as a first step.

The nursing aim

My aim was to make a relationship with Mary. Over the weeks, I heard about her life in and out of care. She had first gone into care when she was aged four, and had been treated in a psychiatric hospital as an adolescent. She was very forgetful a lot of the time, and often forgot to cook for the children. Her drinking was more serious than I had imagined. She continued to feel that Colin was a 'pain' and wanted me to see him, which I agreed to do, but only with her present.

We also planned what she would buy and cook for the family. On one occasion when she came to see me, she said she would have to leave 10 minutes early. She had put a cake in the oven just before leaving home to give to the children when they got in from school. We had spoken about her trying to do this at least once a week. It was interesting that she had done it on the day she came to see me, thus missing out on part of her time with me. It was as if to convince me she was actually doing it, much as a small child might need approval from a parent. Nursing the ego-functioning and inherent strengths in Mary was as important as understanding her underlying fears and anxieties.

She continued to turn up for appointments until I went on leave, and we lost contact for two months. My letters to her home were unanswered, and the family were not on the phone, as we have noted.

I had tried to prepare Mary for my leave and separation from her, knowing her early childhood experience of being left by her mother and placed into care. She, however, could only say that I deserved a holiday and was puzzled why I thought she might miss her time with me, or feel angry that it might seem as if I was dropping her. These issues of transference in my relationship with Mary seemed to be demonstrated most clearly around my holiday breaks.

A chance meeting between the health visitor and Mary in the town led us to know that the family had been evicted from their home because of rent arrears. They were being housed in temporary accommodation, and the health visitor gave me the address. I wrote to say how I had heard the news, and offered an appointment for Mary to come and see me again if she wished. I did not wish to impose myself on the family. It was important to wait for Mary to request my help rather than to 'rescue' her, which, I think, would have reinforced her sense of failure.

She came to see me. She was very angry with the housing department, but denied feeling angry with me. To my mind, however, when I went on holiday, her withdrawal seemed to be a repetition of her childhood response to her mother leaving her.

We all had a fight on our hands to get the family rehoused. There were a lot of rent arrears and, from the housing department's viewpoint, they did not deserve another chance. I learnt that there had been previous evictions.

Some early changes

At this time, the family were living in squalid temporary housing. I had to see them more frequently than usual because of my dealings with the housing department, in order to show them the letters I was sending and to tell them about my phone calls. We agreed between us that Mary would take a back seat over the housing. I would not normally do this, but my taking over the housing issue allowed her not to become an angry child, but to remain an adult and mother to the children.

Mary became more robust during this period. Her physical health improved and the children were at last having proper meals. I saw changes during my home visits; such as a small table and chairs for the children's meals. Derek had given up work and often looked after the children. The children were better dressed, Colin was much more communicative, Nancy became toilet trained, and both Derek and Mary went to an open evening at the school to hear how Colin and Jason were doing. Mary stopped buying them so many toys (which they broke) and spent the money on better food. Derek bought Mary a recipe book. He also started to communicate more with me. They both stopped having such high expectations of the children.

She and Derek were more united than they had been for some time. They were rehoused. Decorating started in earnest, helped by a grant from the DSS. Mary started to take a pride in their home, and the children were starting to blossom. Mary was able to value herself more, although she had not stopped drinking. Colin was no longer sought out as being the difficult child, and had long since stopped soiling. They were all difficult now! Feeding continued to be a focus for our work, but Mary began to feel unwell again and was unable to eat. There were times when we would sit at the kitchen table talking, and she would only have a drink of coffee, and a biscuit if I would eat half of it with her.

How Mary coped with cancer

Around Christmas, she became ill again, and, in January, her general practitioner diagnosed a rare lymphoma of the bone marrow. She was relieved that her symptoms now had a diagnosis, but wondered what a lymphoma of the bone marrow was, and what it would mean for the future. She thought she might only have six months to a year to live, although it is difficult to know where this idea came from. A consultant haematologist and a Macmillan nurse were now involved, and she commenced some oral chemotherapy, although initially she took it erratically. She feared what it was doing to her body and did not want to gain weight.

Mary wanted to see me on her own again at the clinic. She was anxious and confused, said she could not talk about her illness with Derek, and was unsure of what she should tell the children. She told Colin and Jason that she had a mild cancer. She told her extended family and then became mistrustful of the way they rallied around her. She could not feel their concern was genuine, and saw her own mother's concern as being just nosey. In her experience, her mother had never given anything to her freely, either her love or more material things. To this day, she has never asked her mother why she was put into care at four years old, and continues to harbour thoughts she was just 'bad'. Family relationships were always exploitative. The extended family had a system of buying and selling all manner of material goods between each other. Lending money to each other and becoming angry when it was not paid back, seemed to be the currency on which their relationships were maintained. There was always a feeling that no one could be trusted, and everything had to be paid for, including ordinary human favours.

At this time, Mary had dreams of being sucked into a tunnel and not getting out, and of seeing her grandfather in heaven and joining him there. Waking once in the night, she felt terrified, and wrote letters to the children for them to read when she died. She continued to abuse her oral chemotherapy and took two overdoses of antidepressants. She talked about feeling isolated, like a leper in the family. She and Derek were not talking much, and Mary was frightened, and angry that no one had picked up her illness earlier. She was, however, able to share her despair with me, and there was a long period when I carried much of her hopelessness.

Being with Mary

I talked with the staff team to gain support, and to understand my feelings. I also requested extra supervision with the case. Mary was now complaining that Colin was playing up, Jason was having trouble at school, and the girls were being defiant and cheeky. She felt Derek was mollycoddling her, and she had to go along with this to please him, even though she felt it undermined her capabilities. Mary was angry for many weeks. There seemed to be a link between Mary feeling persecuted by Derek and the children, and just how persecuted she must have felt by her cancer.

I heard about the children's behaviour, and could only surmise about how troubled they felt about their mother's deterioration. I suggested to Mary that perhaps the children might benefit from meeting me and a colleague. She refused, saying she would wait and see if things settled down. We had agreed on previous occasions that I would see any of the children if she was worried about them, but I would be led by her on this.

I needed to go on trusting Mary's judgements, while sharing my anxieties with her. She needed to hold on to the autonomy she had found in her relationship with me.

The family's all-pervading sense of loss was, I felt, flooding the family, and me. Mary's own losses were numerous: the loss of the body she once had (she had now gained much weight); the loss of her mind at times, the overdoses, her fantasies about a body invaded by disease; and the loss of the person she was.

She also felt at this time that she had lost her sense of humour. This was shared by Derek, who said in one of our meetings, that she had become a 'pain', which was a poignant moment that struck home about how emotionally painful it all was. For Mary, it seemed easier to think of herself as already dead; thinking about the implications of living, however, helped to shift things again in a positive way.

Mary started attending a local day hospital organized by her Macmillan nurse. It helped to be with others with similar experiences, and she was able to speak about her experience of illness and chemotherapy. Chemotherapy made her feel very ill, but hospital and the hospice cared for her well during these times.

After a long absence, Derek rejoined our meetings. At first, he did not have much to say. He was much more supportive of Mary, and was doing most of the child care. I felt he showed a generosity of spirit in his care for her and the children, but his underlying fears and anxieties were kept at bay. He became involved at the day hospital, doing odd jobs and helping with fund-raising events. The children were also regular visitors there.

Mary told me one day that she felt the hospice was her family now. This was quite a statement from a woman who, two years previously, had told me she would not get close to anybody! It seemed to me that Mary's cancer had given her a legitimate reason to be cared for and had opened up her life in a positive way, which, I suspect, would not have happened had she not become ill. Sexual relations between Mary and Derek began again after many months. Family outings became regular weekend events, with photographs of these trips put in a family album. Mary felt she wanted a record of some happy times for the children, and, rather movingly, she also put her's and Derek's wedding photograph in the back of the album.

Easter brought bad news. Chemotherapy was no longer working, the haematologist and the Macmillan nurse were pessimistic, and bone marrow samples were sent to two leading hospitals in the country for expert advice.

Mary's fears about a bone marrow transplant

My anxieties about Mary led me to meet with her Macmillan nurse. Our discussion revealed feelings of mutual frustration. The nurse and the haematologist had discussed the issue of a bone marrow transplant with Mary. This would give her a better quality of life, but Mary was adamant that she did not want it, and she had not discussed it with me.

When I raised this with Mary, she told me at first that a transplant had never been discussed with her. Then she said that it might have been talked about, but she had not understood what it meant. She then spoke of her very primitive fears that if ever she were to have a transplant it would mean asking a member of her family for bone marrow, and, because they were so unreliable, she would probably be under the anaesthetic waiting for the new marrow, and, whichever family member was donating it would suddenly refuse, perhaps, leaving her to die.

I last saw Mary and Derek and the children some time after our discussion about her fears of transplantation. Mary had subsequently spoken to the consultant haematologist and the Macmillan nurse, and had told them she would consent to whatever treatment they recommended, including a bone marrow transplant if necessary. Our discussion had helped to relieve her fears, and she was so ill that she would try anything to feel better. Mary's sense of humour and straightforwardness pushed their way to the front once more. She had already ordered Derek to give her a crew cut, so that if she lost her hair it would not come as too much of a shock. As for me, Mary thought that if she was admitted for a transplant, I would probably be away on holiday at the time. This was Mary harnessing her sense of humour to make a dig about me being absent at an important time. She sometimes called it 'tit-for-tat', and we used to laugh. At those points, we knew where we stood, in a mutually respecting way.

The nurse–patient relationship is not a uniform professional blueprint, but rather a kaleidoscope of intimacy and distance in some of the most dramatic, poignant and mundane moments of life (Benner, 1984). My relationship with Mary had, I felt, been an important factor in her change process. My awareness of the transference issues helped me to persevere when it seemed that all might be lost. It enabled me to contain the family's feelings of anxiety and aggression until they were ready to face them for themselves. At the time of writing, it is still uncertain what the future will hold for Mary and her family.

References

Benner, P. (1984). *From Novice to Expert: Excellence and Power in Clinical Nursing Practice*. Addison Wesley.
Winnicott, D.W. (1964). *The Family and the Outside World*. Penguin.

Further reading

Simpson, E.A. (1994). Psychological and family centred nursing in the local community. *J. Psychiatr. Mental Health Nurs.*, **2**, 129–130.

Chapter 9
Pain as memory

Gillian Parker

This chapter attempts to explore three things.

First, what happens when abusive experience cannot be recalled? What is the difference between the unmentionable, unspeakable, unthinkable and unbearable? When experience has been so terrible that it is beyond words, even beyond belief, what does this mean to the victim?

Secondly, how does the therapist seek to build a holding structure around such a tortured individual, so that it becomes safer to remember and, more importantly, to refind a sense of self worth?

Thirdly, what is the relationship between pain and imagining? How can the individual, the family, even a nation, survive beyond the barbaric excesses of others, plus their personal defensive excesses, to work towards an interpersonal and group democracy?

The experiences of three women are considered. These are their feelings on looking back, two to childhood experiences, the third to when travelling at 17 years old. Their ability with time to share enough of their experiences to enable them to take positive steps in present-day relationships has perhaps made it worthwhile to remember. To recollect first as bodily pain, then, as the picture became clearer, as flashbacks, which included feeling intense, terrifying moments with all the senses, and then to realize there was someone else there too, the therapist, who was able to bear and share words and memory.

The first account shows the many reasons why words and memory became appallingly crippled, restricted and lost. This is what the patient and I explained to each other. Read of our thinking together about it.

Why words become lost

Trauma involves injuring trust. The word 'trauma' originally meant a 'wound' and, at root, every person exposed to trauma and abuse suffers from the pain of a trust that is wounded, often intentionally, and sometimes irrevocably. Being out of control because one is in the grip of someone else's command introduces a helplessness and a feeling of dependency that feels so terrifying that it can render one speechless. The malevolent intent which is often part of the traumatic equation is so hard to make sense of that the survivor's inner world can become a painful place where flashbacks and memories continue to wreak havoc.

In order to survive the fact that one *has* survived, the human organism deploys an admirable array of defence mechanisms which bring measured relief and a tentative sense of safety. One way of defending oneself against the overwhelming pain of remembering is to stop the memory finding a way into words. Such memories may, instead, be retained in the damaged body tissues themselves. This pain is the language of body memories and follows gross emotional, physical and sexual abuse, or assaults from the outside world. In such circumstances, both trust and the physical body are tortured and the use of words no longer works. The feeling that no-one could bear to hear what has happened is the lonely projection of the survivors who actually feel unable to hear the truth themselves. They may feel literally unable to speak.

To torture originally meant to twist, and abuse of all kinds twists an inner sense of integrity. 'Soul murder' is so hard to live with, both when the abuse is happening and afterwards. It is very difficult to describe. The tragedy of trauma is that it confuses in such a way that all structure, which includes the unifying feeling of integrity, seems to be smashed to bits. The structure of words may also fall apart. Ordinary language is let go. This can be seen in the immediate moments after a shock or accident, when words often become jumbled, or the ability to speak or scream disappears altogether. The more dangerous form of speechlessness is that which comes with sustained abuse, where words can also be actively forbidden by the abuser (who wields enormous power) or in situations where someone has been tortured in such a way that forces us beyond imagination into a place where words have no place. This does not mean there is no language, only that it is not a language of words.

These experiences are felt to be too terrible and too painful to remain in the realm of words. Words, which ordinarily act as meaningful maps for describing feelings and happenings, seem to lose the capacity to contain, and become, instead, weapons in themselves. This is part of why some things are felt to be unspeakable. Words are now dangerous, carrying the power to wound all over again because they are linked to thinking; some experiences of abuse and trauma are so overwhelming that they cannot be thought about afterwards. They have to become unthinkable.

The easiest analogy is to imagine the feeling of having woken from a frightening nightmare, which, no matter how hard one tries, cannot be remembered because the meaning imbued in the dream may be too much to think about. Waking from such a dream is frequently accompanied by a headache or a feeling of physical discomfort. Attention then focuses on the body, which further protects from the fear of the dream. At such times, the ability to think in a way that feels safe is lost; the natural urge is therefore to find a shore, to regain a sense of equilibrium, and the body can act as a metaphorical buoy on which to hold.

How body tissues contain pain

When people have survived a traumatic experience they may need to relegate all knowledge of it to a recess where words do not exist. Surviving the trauma has been enough in itself and for a long time they may feel unable to survive the memories. It has long been recognized that the human organism seems able to erase the fact that something has happened, but it is also known that such happenings do not disappear completely. They merely slip out of view, and much is now understood of how memories can reside out of the reach of consciousness. For instance, memories may also find a repository in the traumatized body tissues themselves, where they are retained, eluding the confines of language because they are felt to be indescribable and, more importantly, unthinkable.

The thought of body tissues as a repository carries within it some helpful ideas. A repository is a safe storehouse, a place of burial, in which a secret can be entrusted. As a defence against being attacked by memory, such a place may be needed to hold the emotional pain in a way that it may be felt as physical pain. Although the physical body memories may be painful in themselves, it is as if this pain is more bearable than ordinary memory. A repository is also a place of preservation. Such memories seem to insist on being preserved, for a time may come when conscious recognition, an approbation of sorts, is needed.

An example of an accident-prone child

This example illustrates the complex combination of how a woman felt unable to know a memory and yet how her physical symptoms persisted in pushing her towards finding the meaning behind her physical pain.

Her eldest brother tried to kill her when she was seven years old, by pushing her from a great height. As she fell, he walked away, leaving her for dead. When help came, she found herself saying that she had fallen and that it was her fault. Her fear of her brother prevented her from feeling able to say what had happened.

Although the injuries were superficial – her broken collar bone and arm healed without any complications – something remained broken inside. For years, this woman would wake from dreaming with a searing pain in her right shoulder, which would click out of place for a few minutes. All she could know of the dreams was of a sensation of falling and she never understood why she felt so shaky about the pain.

It was not until a van drove into the back of her car years later that something stirred in her consciousness from when she was a child. The recent whiplash injury seemed to revive in both memory and body the horror of being forcibly pushed from behind. Fortunately, she was able to talk about why the recent injury was so distressing to her. Pictures of her brother's face came back to her, the sound of his words and laughter as he pushed, and the searing pain of her shoulder dislocating. Finally, it became clear how this body memory was also a 'screen memory' for many similar incidents, which then found their way into words and memories, showing that the relationship with her brother had always been abusive and yet kept so hidden from the family, hidden because she feared first that he would actually kill her if she told, and, secondly, that it might destroy the family if they knew.

The deepest pain was having to face the fact that someone she loved and who was meant to love her had actually hated her enough at times to try to kill her, and that she too hated him for what he had done and had longed for him to die too. It was these thoughts that had been unthinkable. For a long time, it was less painful for her to feel the physical pain in her shoulder at night than to know more.

What this example shows is how essential it is for some memories to emerge in manageable doses, ideally with a feeling of safety and containment around. It is an example of how a psychotherapeutic relationship requires the therapist to go with the client into territory that can feel so dangerous. It also shows how body memories may also be protecting abusive family systems. Such systems survive by the rule of the most violent kind of silence, refusing to hear what is really going on and by silencing any attempt at disclosure. It is understandable that words then become useless. It is as if the human organism resorts to the much earlier functions of the brain, not as a linguistic and memory bank, but as a signaller and storer of primarily physical sensations and needs. Signals of distress are being sent out by body memories. It brought immense relief, in this case, to find the links and meanings held in the physical symptoms, but the sadness of understanding was also felt as great grief.

Body memories as a painful protection

It is essential to keep in mind both the protective value and the cost of defence mechanisms. Body memories are an example of how complicated the costs and benefits of defences can be. They are expensive, but they may also cost less than knowing too much too soon, for some memories are too much and can make one feel like dying all over again. There are times in abusive situations when death seems preferable and less cruel than life. This is why body memories should be explored with great caution, and with plenty of time, and only when there is a holding situation around metaphorically to hold the individual, who may feel that the emotional and physical being is falling apart.

The paradox about body memories is that they seem actually to help one *not* remember in words, whilst simultaneously reminding that something feels very wrong. This paradoxical mixed message is important and well described by Judith Lewis Herman (1992) in *Trauma and Recovery:*

> The conflict between the will to deny horrible events and the will to proclaim them aloud is the central dialectic of psychological trauma . . . The story of the traumatic event surfaces not as a verbal narrative but as a symptom.

The symptoms we are specifically concerned with are physical, which have a peculiar persistence and which seem to be saying something in a language all of their own. There are many different kinds of body memories and many different origins for them. Here the focus is on the body memories that come in the aftermath of trauma and abuse. The hypothesis is that the mature thinking and remembering brain, which we rely on to help us to make sense of situations, can actually be so overwhelmed by the combined impact of emotional and physical trauma that it resorts to a more pre-verbal form of functioning in order to help someone to survive. Somehow, the physical body itself, the tissues and cells, become the focus of activity, and links between sensation and thought are severed. For some, the pain of abuse, particularly if it is prolonged and involves people who are meant to be trusted, is so great because nothing seems to make any sense any more, and the twisted and mixed messages which they are forced to take inside themselves perpetuate a feeling of spiralling insecurity inside. One way of trying to stabilize such chaos is to fix feeling into the physical body, as an anchor.

An example of a child overwhelmed

The dynamic interplay between mind, body and emotions is blatantly apparent in an abusive situation, as this example shows.

If a father is imposing his sexual demands on his daughter, there is the combination of his losing control of his emotional impulses, which he then channels through his body into his child. At first, his body contains his feelings but he then uses his body to push those feelings into the child, both physically and emotionally penetrating her sense of self. The child then responds with her own feelings, as well as being filled with the adult's feelings. The body tissues are damaged and feel pain.

The culmination is that the brain is overwhelmed with an influx of painful information; messages of pain come from both the sensory nerve endings in the body tissues and the sensitivity of the emotional nerves. Although usually a master at making sense of situations, at such times the brain itself is being asked to make sense of feelings and pain which seem to lack structure for the simple reason that a central tenet of trust has been shattered and replaced with confusion.

This example of a woman whose father had used her as a sexual partner for many years shows further the futility of ever trying completely to separate emotional and physical feelings. Although much of this memory still remains a hazy blur, she was able eventually to describe a recurrent pain in her neck and shoulders which would come on when she felt pressurized. The pain felt like 'fingerprints', as if a large hand was gripping her. Even finding these words made her feel unbearable fear and, when asked, she started to talk of how her father would use that same grip to push her head down when he wanted oral sex. She resisted by pushing her neck up against his hand, which then just pushed down harder, with increasing excitement on his part; no words were ever said. This happened many times, over years.

What is relevant here is that it was the combination of the feel of his fingers in the body tissues plus his desire and lack of caring for her own feelings which made the whole scenario so impregnated with feelings and thoughts which she could not bear to remember. However, her neck never forgot, nor, in her heart, did she. As I write, she can still only find words up to the point when the grip is pushing her down. If she tries to say more of what happened next she becomes overwhelmed with a choking nausea and starts wanting to be sick as if to reassure herself that she need never feel forced to swallow such bodily fluids and circumstances again. It is as if the sensory nerve endings in her neck, mouth and stomach are still replaying the feelings felt during the actual abuse.

External trauma as a biological and emotional shock

One of the most distressing aspects of trauma is that someone is forced to feel overwhelmed. Whether this occurs in physical or sexual abuse, in situations of torture, or in an accident, one common denominator is a feeling of helplessness in the presence of an external person or power which seems capable of (and at times fixed on) shattering one's existence.

Psychoanalysis and psychotherapy have been forced to pay increasing attention to the damage inflicted by an injurious external world and what this then does to one's inner world. Charles Rycroft (1985) highlights the importance of recognizing the damage of trauma:

> There exists, however, a type of occurrence in which sensations are forced upon consciousness and the psyche which it has no option but to perceive, but which it is equally unable to assimilate and convert into experiences of a meaningful, let alone enriching, kind. These are the sensations produced by traumatic events, that is by unexpected disasters such as earthquakes, car or plane accidents, or sexual or other physical violations. The immediate effect of such experiences is a state of shock, in which the victim is unable to comprehend what has happened to him. Such events are experiences in the sense that the occurrence thereafter forms part of his biography, but are not experiences in the sense that they acquire meaning or significance for him. He may, if he is lucky, get over it, but he will not have been enriched by it. Memories of traumatic events are more like foreign bodies embedded in the psyche than essential parts of it, since they remain disconnected from the continuum of experience.

What Rycroft seems to be stressing is that trauma is, at first, conscious, and is then necessarily 'forgotten' but is never, to quote him again, 'a true part of the psyche', quite different from memories, wishes and emotions, which have been disowned or repressed without the involvement of external trauma. This is why, ultimately, memories of trauma do insist on surfacing. Herman (1992) says of this:

> Equally as powerful as the desire to deny atrocities is the conviction that denial does not work . . . Remembering and telling the truth about terrible events are pre-requisites both for the restoration of social order and for the healing of individual victims . . . When the truth is finally recognized, survivors can begin their recovery.

The difficulty is that such stories are not only hard to tell but also hard to hear. This is why it is essential at times to ask about symptoms and not always to wait for someone to tell, for the survivor of abuse feels already that no one really wants to hear. Herman warns that 'all too commonly neither patient nor therapist recognises the link between the presenting problem and the history of chronic trauma'. There is, however, increasing reason to hope that this is changing.

Therapists of many different professions know from watching and listening to the survivors of trauma how dynamic is the link between mind, body and emotions, but it is reassuring to find scientific research acknowledging the connections too. It is interesting that, in *The Oxford Companion to the Mind* (Gregory, 1987), there is an entry under 'Pain' which says:

> Recent evidence, however, shows that pain is not simply a function of the amount of bodily damage alone, but is influenced by attention, anxiety, suggestion, prior experience, and other psychological variables (Melzack and Wall, 1982) . . . The psychological and neurological data, then, force us to reject the concept of a single straight through sensory transmission system. In recent years the evidence on pain has moved in the direction of recognising the plasticity and modifiability of events in the central nervous system. Pain is a complex perceptual and affective experience determined by the unique past history of the individual, by the meaning to him of the injurious agent or situation and by his 'state of mind' at the moment, as well as by the sensory nerve patterns evoked by physical stimulation.

Much of this chapter requires the reader to let go of the language of logic in order to be able to listen to what *cannot* be said, to listen to the space, as it were, in order to find meaning in the language of body symptoms and feelings. There is, however, an analogy within the basic biological structure of the body, which is useful.

In *Studies on Hysteria*, Breuer and Freud (1893–1895) have much to say about the link between physical reactions and sensations and unconscious memory, leading to the well-known hypothesis that 'hysterics suffer mainly from reminiscences'. There is a particularly poignant paragraph, which appeals directly to our discussion here. Having described physical symptoms occurring in the wake of thought, Breuer says:

> It would be plausible to believe that, though the symptoms in question were ideogenic in the first instance, the repetition of them has, to use Romberg's phrase (1840), 'imprinted' them into the body, and they would now no longer be based on a psychical process but on modifications in the nervous system which have occurred in the meantime: they would have become self-sufficient, genuinely somatic symptoms.

In cases involving trauma, the term 'ideogenic' can be replaced with 'traumatogenic', for it is the external trauma which then becomes the unthinkable thought.

Remembering smells is an obvious example of how the stimulation of the olfactory nerves can evoke either a physiological or an emotional reaction. Observation suggests that body memories are intricately involved with the central nervous system and the endocrine system. The nervous system helps to control and integrate (giving rise to a feeling of physical integrity, which adds to or diminishes a feeling of emotional integrity) all body activities by sensing changes, interpreting them, and reacting to them.

The nerve impulse is the body's quickest way of controlling and maintaining homoeostasis, which is linked with a feeling of emotional equilibrium. Body memories frequently involve pain and so the hypothesis is that the nervous system is being stimulated by a memory that is far from the reach of consciousness.

In *An Introduction to the Human Body*, Gerard Tortora (1988) describes nerve impulses and what he says about the myelinated 'A' fibres seems very relevant:

> The A fibres are located in the axons of large sensory nerves that relay impulses associated with touch, pressure, position of joints, heat, and cold. They are also found in all motor nerves that convey impulses to the skeletal muscles. Sensory A fibres generally connect the brain and spinal cord with sensors that detect danger in the outside environment. Motor A fibres stimulate the muscles that can do something about the situation. If you touch a hot object, information about the heat passes over sensory A fibres to the spinal cord. There it is relayed to motor A fibres that stimulate the muscles of the hand to withdraw instantaneously. The A fibres are located where split-second reaction may mean survival.

Further exploration of the biological reactions within the body are beyond the scope of this chapter, but what stands out in bold relief is that the body and emotions work together with a wonderful wisdom simply to keep a person alive. Body memories are no different. Although so distressing in themselves, they seem to allow unthinkable thoughts and unspeakable messages to be memorized as a way of protecting someone from being overwhelmed again by being exposed to conscious memories and words. The defences resorted to can be Draconian but, on the whole, they work for survival, and this is where the relief in interpreting body memories and finding a language of meaning lies.

An example of how body and memory refused to die

The third example shows how a woman's body symptoms actively tried to prevent her from sleeping. Although exhausting, this was actually protective because her sleep was full of nightmares (which she was unable to remember) but which made her feel terrified and out of control.

This feeling of being out of control was the very feeling she could not bear when she was held for over 24 hours, at knifepoint, by a madman. During this ordeal, she was raped vaginally and anally many times and forced to do things which she still cannot describe. Having been left alive, she vowed to place all conscious memory of those hours in a coffin and bury it deep within herself and out of reach. However, she still carried this coffin within and after several years she was forced to listen to the increasing sound of her physical symptoms: recurrent discharges and infections, back pain, and the protective symptom, sleeplessness. At night, on getting into bed, her rectal muscles would go into spasms which would throw her into acute physical pain and prevent sleep. She would not allow herself to think of links, or of what this pain might be. She simply experienced it, just as she had had to experience the original torture during which her muscles had also fought against giving into the man's physical demands. Now, with the help of hindsight, she feels the spasms were trying to remind her that she had tried to resist (even though the resistance was overwhelmed) and to ask her to seek some help about why the night was so terrifying. The thought of help was terrifying in itself, for it would mean digging up the metaphorical coffin and asking someone to look inside with her. It also necessitated the therapist watching her through her sleep to understand this very private communication of pain.

With time, enough trust was built up for us to look together into the coffin and see the very damaged body kept inside for what it was. It was somewhat like the moving image of Mary holding the damaged body of

Jesus after being taken down from the cross, to honour and then to grieve for the terrible things that human beings can do to one another. It was also important to affirm that the patient's body never died: it was just forced to give in.

When integrity is injured

Can you envisage the sensory nerve endings being abused in a way that makes no sense to an individual's sense of integrity? With external abuse, they send a message to the brain, which interprets the message as pain, but the brain too has to cope with the horror of the happening. The brain now instructs the motor neurons to respond. It is important to notice that motor neurons are also called 'association neurons', for it is at this point where, in body memories, there is a great attempt to sever all further conscious associations. To cope with the lack of sense, the brain can also instruct the motor neurons to respond inappropriately. For example, the body may freeze when movement is needed.

It may seem strange to describe how distressing physical memories may actually be trying to help and protect, and why they seem compelled to recur, sometimes over decades. Gregory Bateson (1972) had a special interest in the idea of unity between mind and body and, as a biologist, had some important ideas about both. In *Steps to an Ecology of Mind*, he compares the compulsion to repeat painful situations or feelings with an escalating positive feedback process:

> It will be noted that the possible existence of such a positive feedback loop, which will cause a runaway in the direction of increasing discomfort up to some threshold (which might be on the other side of death), is not included in conventional theories of learning. But a tendency to verify the unpleasant by seeking repeated experience of it is a common human trait.

Body memories may persist and recur in an effort to tempt the sufferer to seek help. It is doubly tragic when the help sought ends by increasing a feeling of isolation, but it is still worth applauding the motive of the physical symptom. The aftermath of the rape ordeal described above resulted in recurrent gynaecological infections which resisted antibiotics as if determined to maintain a discharge. The link between emotional distress and the suppression of the immune system is now well known (Coe, et al. 1985), so it is not surprising that this woman should have a lowered physical resistance, which correlated with her lowered resistance to face the world. What had greater meaning to her, however, was how her body persisted in having discharges, particularly in a menstrual flow which would last nearly all month, almost as a form of weeping in a way she herself could not. Her symptoms meant she had to keep seeking help; eventually she found the right help.

How destruction from outside can lead to longings to self-destruct or die

In finding a positive purpose for body memories, it is important not to deny the distress they can cause. The people in the examples had all at times longed to die so as not to feel their bodies. The important point is that they did not want to die to escape memories or flashbacks, but to escape the living and feeling body. Instead, various ways of damaging the body were used. Feelings of punishment, control, relief and despair were all intermingled, whether the wounds inflicted were cuts, starvation or sleep deprivation. One could hardly bear to eat because the process of digesting caused physical sensations that provoked feelings of panic. These feelings of panic did not start to ease until she was able to link them to happenings during her 24-hour ordeal. Although she is still unable to speak about those memories, she has at least been able to experience them with someone else present and this has been very important to her.

Another more distressing function of body memories may be linked to the increased release of endogenous opiates during stress. In *From Pain to Violence*, Felicity de Zulueta (1993) describes the relevance of the opioid system:

> Van der Kolk (1989) notes that one of the prime functions of the infant–mother relationship is to modulate physiological arousal in the infant. This is probably achieved through the opioid system.

This is relevant to the feelings of unbearable anxiety experienced by those who have been tortured, for de Zulueta goes on to quote Van der Kolk: 'These victimised people neutralise their hyperarousal by a variety of addictive behaviours including compulsive re-exposure to situations reminiscent of the trauma.' De Zulueta then says:

> This important finding casts a new light on the phenomenon of repetition compulsion: trauma victims may well become addicted to their trauma, recreating it in some form or other throughout their lives. The repeated exposure to traumatic stress produces both the need for the activation of the

endogenous opioid system and the resultant withdrawal symptoms. This may partly explain the link between childhood abuse and self-destructive behaviour: often these people become self-mutilators; many report finding peace and relief from their pain and arousal in the act of cutting themselves.

It is only through the experiences of traumatized people who can actually speak and find words that more can be known and understood about how pain is memorized. Psychological research published in the late 1970s made important forays into this distressing area. De Zulueta also talks of this:

> Recent psychological research shows that the retrieval of information is, in part, dependent on reinstituting the brain context that was present when the to-be-remembered event was encoded and stored in memory (Weingartner, et al. 1977). It is also in keeping with the postulated existence of a variety of 'memory banks' in the brain; this means that different sets of memories and their affective components can coexist in the mind, one being unavailable or unconscious to the other (Gazzangia and Le Doux, 1978).

I would add only that the affective components can also coexist in the body tissues as well.

Having talked with these patients, I have felt that the body can relinquish whatever repetitive pain is occurring: if the biological and emotional intercellular spaces can be filled with a good enough feeling of trust with a psychotherapist; if, then, a way can be found to coax the memories to learn to find words as a way of leaving the tissues and cells; and if the person who has suffered can begin to test out that these memories can be survived by both himself or herself and the person they tell. Until such a setting is available, it is better by far to let the body cry, shout and scream, than force a mind and spirit to succumb to being overwhelmed all over again, for this may not be survivable.

Body memories have a sense, a safety and a security, for traumatized or abused people often have no internal representation of another person that feels secure. The body is the closest, most trustworthy object they have, even though they may simultaneously loathe it, simply because it was present during the abuse. The isolation is acute. Herman (1992) describes this:

> Whatever new identity she develops in freedom must include the memory of her enslaved self. Her image of her body must include a body that can be controlled and violated. Her image in relation to others must include a person who can lose and be lost to others.

Restoring communication between body memories and the mind and emotions is a painstaking task for both therapist and client, but it is possible. The search for a mutual language that makes sense of what had lost sense is a starting point for beginning to live again, rather than just surviving.

Collating, understanding and interpreting

What is most important is an understanding of the essential defence mechanisms that traumatized people need. Interpretations have always drawn, often covertly, on bodily information gathered by the senses as well as intellectual energy and verbal communication.

In all these examples, at some point, the interpretation might have been seen as a translation from observed body language into words within a good enough holding situation. This was seen, for example, when the sufferer sat in silence, unable to speak, one hand over her mouth representing the forceful assailant, whilst her stomach muscles went into repetitive spasms. Often, what was described as an interpretation was a 'fractile' (an encapsulated mime) of the actual abuse, with both the role of victim and of the perpetrator indicated.

At some point, there was also a realization of being overwhelmed, where the intervention had to have the quality of lifting a confused, distressed and terrified child out of an overwhelming and damaging situation and forming a protective setting. Equally, there were occasions when, to help shimmering attempts at trust, transitional objects needed to be exchanged: things to take away, break, mend and repair. Eventually these could be seen as the outward evidence of an inner gain, a replacement introject.

At the Inner City Centre in the City of London, where I work, therapy has been important, but just as important has been the sensitivity and wisdom that comes with the people seeking help; it may be personal, family or cultural. With support, they start using their own sensitivity and wisdom again. This has been particularly so with people like the three who have helped me with this chapter.

Often the story is more complicated. For instance, imagine these cases had not been three, but one, in which a childhood had been very bad and young adult life too; imagine if a mother had been raped as well as her daughter.

The rewarding experience is that people make extraordinary use of some of the therapy. A mother and grandmother may be helped by the patient, or mother may start having a new-found way of being aware of how her children are feeling, and thoughts of how to safeguard and look out for grandchildren can become possible.

Pain and imagination have recoupled to reconstruct. Experience can be learned and repetitive behaviours replaced by flexibility. Boundaries and rights are recognized. Life can be negotiated. We feel that the fact that because one person has found a way safely to spiral backwards, there is the personal possibility of spiralling forward, knowing that others may be the better protected; the spiral has the feel of a safer future.

Summary

The uncovering of the structure of torture and its ability to destroy the person and the artefacts of family life shows that it is experienced as so soul-destroying that initially it necessitates losing the ability to recall in words. In the place of words, a 'false self' is developed and a fictional, although shared, reality is created to bridge beyond destruction, silencing alternative reality.

The violence of this silence becomes a totalitarian force, which further victimizes the individual, although it may preserve the group. What is also sacrificed is the internal integrity of the organization.

In therapy, there is a difficult move from the false self's fictional reality back to the now shared horrors and pain, and then gradually to rebuilding relationships which, although far from perfect, are at best ordinarily good enough, and contain much wisdom, kindliness and drive.

As a testimony to the experiences recounted here, and to all those who feel the pain of body memories, I turn to Philip Vellacott's (1963) words about the conflict between life and warmth and the processes of civilized man:

> . . . the universe is not on the side of civilisation; and . . . a life combining order with happiness is something men must win for themselves in continual struggle with an unsympathetic environment.

The abusive environment is certainly unsympathetic and the struggle to reclaim a right to order and happiness seems to become possible with the coupling of pain and imagination. It is this that is the important step to reconstruction and, finally, to creativity.

Acknowledgements

To people who also work beyond words, who have shown me much: the therapeutic communities of the Cassel Hospital, the Henderson Hospital and the Mulberry Bush School; Gabrielle Parker, psychotherapist and dance and movement therapist; Jennifer Fasal, masseuse, director of POPAN (Prevention of Professional Abuse Network); and especially to Amanda Jones, working with children and their families in pain in the paediatric department of the King George's Hospital, Ilford, Essex.

References

Bateson, G. ed. (1972). The cybernetics of 'self': a theory of alcoholism. In *Steps to an Ecology of Mind*, p. 328, Chandler.

Breuer, J. and Freud, S. (1893–1895). *Hypnoid States: Studies on Hysteria*, p. 299, Penguin.

Coe, C.L., Wiener, S.G., Rosenberg, L.T. and Levine, S. (1985). Endocrine and immune responses to separation and maternal loss in nonhuman primates. In *The Psychobiology of Attachment and Separation* (M. Reite and T. Field, eds.) pp. 163–199, Academic Press.

Gazzangia, M.S. and Le Doux, J.E. (1978). *The Split Brain and the Integrated Mind*. Plenum Press.

Gregory, R.L. ed. (1987). *The Oxford Companion to The Mind*, pp. 574–575, Oxford University Press.

Herman, J.L. (1992). *Trauma and Recovery*. Basic Books.

Melzack, R. and Wall, P.D. (1982). *The Challenge of Pain*. Penguin.

Romberg, M.H. (1840). *Lehrbuch der Nervenkrankheiten des Menschen*, p. 229, Berlin.

Rycroft, C. (1985). *Psychoanalysis and Beyond*, p. 163, Hogarth Press.

Tortora, G.J. (1988). *An Introduction to the Human Body*, p. 181, Harper and Row.

Van der Kolk, B.A. (1989). The compulsion to repeat the trauma: re-enactment, revictimisation and masochism. *Psychiatr. Clin. North Am.*, 12, 389–411.

Vellacott, P. (1963). Foreword to translation of Euripedes. In *Medea and Other Plays*, (P. Vellacott, translator) p. 9, Penguin.

Weingartner, H., Miller, H. and Murphy, D.L. (1977). Mood-state dependent retrieval of verbal associations. *J. Abnorm. Psychol.*, 86, 276–284.

Zulueta, F. de (1993) *From Pain to Violence: the Traumatic Roots of Destructiveness*. Whurr.

Chapter 10

Knowing patients: how much and how well?

Louise de Raeve

The focus of this chapter is on general nursing; different considerations may apply in psychiatry. In ordinary encounters with people, we seem to distinguish between knowing a lot about a person, for example, via someone's employment record or through social gossip, and knowing them in the sense that one might speak of knowing a friend. However, it would be odd if, in claiming to know a person, one did not also know a considerable amount about them. Thus, perhaps one can say that knowing much about a person is a necessary but not a sufficient condition of knowing a person well. Both senses of knowing a person may rely on observation and dialogue, but, while I could come to know a lot about a person through dialogue with third parties or the reading of diaries and memoirs, I cannot claim to know a person well unless I am or have been in direct engagement with him or her.

Nurses can certainly claim, with justification, to know their patients on both accounts. We sometimes know a lot about people in the informational sense and we certainly see it as part of our job to have some sort of relationship with our patients, such that we can claim to know them in the second sense, albeit in a limited way. Rarely, however, would we say we knew a patient well. When we do say this, it is perhaps meant more usually to imply that, as far as knowing patients goes generally, we know this person well, but this is not to be confused with what we might mean by knowing a friend well.

Boundaries

Indeed, it has become a requirement of a good nurse to try and get to know her patients. (For the purposes of this chapter, 'the nurse' will be referred to by the feminine pronoun and 'the patient' by the masculine.)

Salvage (1990) refers to this as the 'new nursing' and links it with the development of primary nursing where emphasis is placed on 'individualized' and 'holistic' care. Current changes in nurse education have enhanced this trend. When put crudely, the idea seems to be that the more the nurse knows her patient, in both senses of knowing, the better placed she will be to nurse him. However, it is not intended that this knowing should be unlimited, for no one seriously proposes that boundaries are not important. Engagement may be important but so also is the maintenance of a degree of distance and objectivity, which is essential for both the nurse and the patient in order for nursing to occur. This necessity of boundaries strongly suggests that, in nursing, our need to know patients is primarily for the purpose of helping people to get better, and that we only need to know them to that extent. However, this 'extent' cannot be predetermined and will vary from individual to individual, so, even to make this assessment, would require rudimentary knowledge of the person.

One can make clear the purposive nature of a nurse's need to know her patients by considering the case of a person who is admitted for minor surgery, who makes a speedy recovery and is discharged after two days. In such a situation, no nurse would say that the treatment was a success except for the fact that there was no time to develop a relationship with the patient! In taking this view, it does not mean that all nurses' conversations with patients are conducted in an instrumental spirit along the lines of: 'I am only talking to you for a purpose.' This would be grossly to distort much of the natural and spontaneous conversation that takes place between nurses and patients. Perceiving nurse–patient communications as purposive in general does not prevent individual interchanges from being seen as valuable in themselves.

Considerable thought has been given in nursing to the question of what constitutes an appropriate boundary when it comes to matters of what nurses should or should not do with patients and how to manage a situation if either party becomes too attached to the other, so that the professional nature of the relationship threatens to be lost in confusion. Less, however, has been said about what might be an appropriate boundary for the gathering of information about patients. This is not a question of how such information should be shared or stored, which raises all the well-known issues of confidentiality, but a prior question of what needs to be asked and why, and whether such lines of enquiry are morally justifiable. The moral justification (or lack of it) will hinge upon a comparison between those morally valuable states or conditions which may be infringed by such enquiries and the necessity of gathering such information to fulfil other morally worthy aims.

Three perspectives

When I was working in a hospital occupational health department, one of my main jobs was to carry out medical examinations for staff who were about to be employed. I was new to the work and thus tended to do things by the letter in an attempt to do a good job and get things right. One day I was doing a medical for a would-be student nurse and on my form was a question separate from that of: 'How many children do you have?', which asked about numbers of pregnancies. I duly asked all the questions on my form and, when it came to the pregnancy question, the prospective student nurse burst into tears, saying she had not thought anyone would ever ask her that. She had had an abortion in the past. It is not clear whether or not being asked such a question was a damaging experience for this student, for I did not confirm her fear that she would be judged for this part of her past and we decided that I would write nothing about it on the form.

Why was it even necessary to ask the question? When I spoke to the senior occupational health nurse about this episode, she said that, in fact, she never asked that question, in which case there was an organizational problem of a gap between what the paperwork demanded and the moral and clinical discretion being exercised by individuals. There had presumably been no collective thinking for some time about what was needed and why.

The second and third perspectives come from the literature. Marc Girard (1988) has some arresting things to say about medicine, which I think apply equally to nursing. He talks about psychoanalysis and the taboo against any sexual relationship in such an encounter, and concludes that bodily privacy is essential for psychiatric patients and emotional privacy for medical or surgical patients. Girard claims that patients should not be asked to 'surrender both psychically and physically: one or the other must be chosen'. He observes (p. 28) that the fundamental question of medical ethics becomes: ' . . . how to establish with precision the *distance* to which a patient is entitled in order to feel respected and recognised?' He goes on to refer to the patient's 'autonomy' and 'right to privacy'.

The third perspective concerns the comments Carl May (1993) makes regarding his research into nurse–patient relationships. He notes that, if values change concerning what constitutes good nursing, so inevitably will the criteria change for determining 'good' (co-operative) as opposed to 'bad' (unco-operative) patients. His claim is that the connection between these ideas is stronger than a merely contingent association. May (p. 186) observes that:

> Because 'knowing' patients and 'involvement' are so intimately linked, the patient who will not permit herself to be known and with whom 'talk' cannot be conducted represents an obstacle to the kinds of nursing practice informed by the imperative towards a non-bureaucratic and individualized encounter.

In the new nursing system, May (p. 189) claims that:

> The individual patient, therefore, has a responsibility to accept individual care: and just as the patient who fails to co-operate with the care of the body is held responsible for his or her actions, the patient who resists or obstructs the nurse's attempts to formulate a personal relationship in which self-revelation may be performed is open to judgement about the extent to which they are to blame for this.

What all three illustrations demonstrate is that, while one might want in general to embrace this new nursing, one might need to be circumspect in considering appropriate limits to what we need to know about patients. A cynic could claim that this psychosocial approach to care is merely a nursing attempt to carve out our own unique territory, away from medical eyes and medical control. Thus, it could be claimed that these changes have nothing much to do with what is good for patients and everything to do with what is good for nursing as a profession. However, while clearly critical of some aspects of the new nursing approach, neither Salvage (1990) nor May (1992, 1993, 1995) hold such a cynical view. Both acknowledge that there is evidence to suggest that, in general, patients gain from a more personal approach to their care. May (1993: p. 182) says: ' . . . "good" interpersonal relationships between staff and patients appeared to contribute significantly to recovery rates . . . ', and Salvage (1990: p. 43) considers that research studies support the 'impression that ONDU [Oxford Nursing Development Unit] provided good quality care using methods which merit further scrutiny'.

The significance of privacy

This challenge of a need for further scrutiny will be pursued but not empirically. It seems to me that one of the issues the new nursing has hitherto failed to address adequately is the significance of the patient's privacy to nurse–patient relationships. Girard (1988) refers to the patient's 'right to privacy'. This is not a new idea to nursing, for we are properly and continuously conscious of pulling round bedside curtains, closing toilet doors and so forth, but I do not think we have given much thought to the need to respect, and perhaps even protect, the patient's privacy by the kinds of questions we ask and the sort of verbal information we think we need to know as nurses.

Philosophically, there is no agreement about exactly what privacy is and why it is important, but, as Fried (1984: p. 209) points out: 'Privacy is not simply an absence of information about us in the minds of others; rather it is the *control* we have over information about ourselves.' He goes on to observe that it would be ironic merely to speak of the privacy of a 'lonely man on a desert island', which is a point that brings out the relational context of privacy. Privacy is important to us because we are social creatures with a public life.

In a similar vein, Derlega and Chaikin (1977: p. 103) adopt Altman's (1975) definition of privacy as being an '*interpersonal boundary process* by which a person or group regulates interaction with others', and they consider that this process of control defines personal identity by contributing to one's sense of autonomy and self-worth and by emphasizing one's uniqueness and individuality (p. 113). If one grants these ideas, one must conclude that, at the very least, privacy is necessary for the preservation and growth of a person's sense of integrity: his sense of physical, moral, emotional and spiritual intactness.

Let us consider these ideas in the light of the example I gave at the beginning of this chapter about the prospective student nurse having her pre-employment medical examination. It was my territory and not hers. She needed to pass her medical to take up a chosen career and I was a gatekeeper. I was the one asking personal questions and this was not expected to be reciprocal. It seems to me that to ask highly personal questions (whether justifiable or not) is a serious invasion of privacy because, in the nature of the power relations that exist, people are to some extent compromised in their ability to defend themselves. In addition, the invasiveness may be increased by the emotional valency of the question, of which the questioner may or may not be aware. In my particular illustration, the prospective student nurse had no defence available to her because, even if she had wanted to lie, my question tapped directly into her painful memories such that tears came before she had a chance to think. It could certainly be said that I had a duty to respect this student's privacy, out of regard for her vulnerability and my power.

Nevertheless, an acknowledged claim to a right of privacy and an agreed duty to protect it may not be binding in any absolute sense. If, instead of being in occupational health, I had been a midwife in an antenatal clinic and the student nurse a pregnant woman coming for checkups, the need to know would probably outweigh the need to respect the privacy of a person's obstetric history, although, of course, a degree of respect can still be shown in the way such information is gained.

Similarly, while a person's history of loss and bereavement is no business of anybody for admission to a surgical ward, unless the patient chooses to make it so, such information may be quite crucial to the treatment of a person admitted to a psychiatric unit in a state of severe depression. The context, thus, seems to be determinative of the moral weight that will be given to protecting privacy or legitimating enquiry regarding specific issues. This begins to make it seem as if privacy can simply be waived if something more compelling comes along. This leads into a philosophical disagreement about precisely how important privacy is and why.

Why is privacy important?

According to Williams (1990: p. 223), some writers such as Wellman (1978) seem to think that privacy is important merely because of all the advantages it seems to produce. For example, it preserves one's sense of security and one's liberty from state intervention and it is essential for the maintenance of extremely important human relationships. In other words, it has instrumental value. However, as Williams (p. 225) observes, if you take this view in isolation, 'it may be possible to speak of *trading* some or indeed all those advantages for others, perhaps, for example, less privacy in exchange for a higher standard of living'.

In the above examples, this is indeed what we seem to be doing. We manifest less respect for privacy when other moral concerns such as the proper care of patients seem more compelling. Indeed, in the case of special clinics, the public control of venereal disease and the interests of third parties are seen to justify very invasive questions for the purpose of contact tracing.

If this instrumental vision of privacy (the idea that its value lies in the ends it serves) was all that mattered, it would be easy for nurses to claim that respecting privacy merely required refraining from asking invasive questions without careful moral scrutiny for the necessity of doing so, and that, when justifiable, such questions should be asked with sensitivity. Would this be enough? My suggestion is that we actually need to do more, that a crucial aspect of nursing requires that we should see ourselves as needing actively to protect a patient's privacy and that this extends beyond the drawing of curtains and the shutting of doors, to protection from invasive inquiries and from our own curiosity. It may even entail helping a patient to refrain from disclosure.

To support this view, I draw upon those philosophical writers who have suggested that privacy does not merely have instrumental value. Fried (1984: p. 205) for example, says:

> It is my thesis that privacy is not just one possible means among others to insure some other value, but that it is necessarily related to ends and relations of the most fundamental sort: respect, love, friendship and trust. Privacy is not merely a good technique for furthering these fundamental relations; rather without privacy they are simply inconceivable. They require a context of privacy or the possibility of privacy for their existence.

Williams (1990: p. 224) says:

> My argument is that the ethical significance of our need for privacy is an essential feature of our nature as moral selves, so that if the need for privacy should diminish or disappear, then our nature as moral selves will alter as well. Furthermore, having control over certain kinds of information about ourselves is a condition of the moral integrity we may possess, an integrity which can only be maintained through our own agency.

These statements reflect the previously quoted statement of Derlega and Chaikin (1977), but they introduce a different emphasis. The claim now is that far from privacy 'contributing' to and 'emphasizing' autonomy, self-worth and integrity, privacy is related to these concepts in such an essential way that not only would such concepts be weakened by the nonexistence of privacy, they would be eroded. This seems to suggest an internal relationship between privacy and these other values, and to indicate that privacy has moral value in itself as well as in relation to the good states of affairs that it is seen to promote. If this view is accepted, it does not imply that it would never be morally justifiable to compromise privacy in favour of some more pressing moral concern, but it adds moral weight to the notion of privacy which is missing in a purely instrumental interpretation. Both Fried and Williams have arguments to support their positions. I want, however, to assume the validity of this way of thinking about privacy and consider what might be its consequences for nursing.

Nursing, privacy and integrity

Generally speaking, the empowerment view of nursing that accompanies notions of individualized care of patients is that, while we may need temporarily to take over many caring activities that people cannot do for themselves, we should always be mindful of the need to hand back this function as soon as possible. Proper mindfulness in this respect determines how the taking over will, in fact, be done. In a psychological and physical sense, we also have to understand how much the experience of illness threatens a person's sense of integrity. Oliver Sacks (1986: p. 122) draws attention to this when writing about his own illness: 'When I felt physically helpless, immobile, confined, I felt morally helpless, paralysed, contracted, confined – and not just contracted, but contorted as well, into roles and postures of abjection.'

It is certainly a nursing responsibility not to add to this predicament but to try where possible to help to restore integration. The sensitive work of a stoma-care nurse or a nurse working with a new amputee is all about this kind of reintegration of body and psyche, such that a patient can feel properly autonomous on departure. Here is one account of this process:

> I can remember the first day Naomi [the patient] massaged her stump. She was so tentative. She was frightened of touching it. So, I just took her through a few basic massage techniques, and said: 'It's really nice if you just give it a rub, like this . . . ' You could see her during the day: the circles were getting bigger and bigger, and more firm, and the hands and the stump were an item. It wasn't a stump that she was barely touching. It was beautiful, the way you could see it happening (Taylor, 1993: p. 36).

How might we be able to capture a similar kind of delicacy and sensitivity in nursing in relation to the protection of a patient's sense of privacy, while at the same time trying to know the person sufficiently to be able to nurse well?

My own partial answer to this question is to look at what happens in the nursing care of premature neonates. What is striking about such a context is that, here, nursing care is provided for a new human life about whom, by definition, there is no prior knowledge of the person to be gained and in relation to whom no other party, such as the parents, can shed any historical light, beyond facts about the baby's birth. No past psychosocial information can be gleaned by asking questions of anybody and yet nurses are not irredeemably handicapped in such a context, far from it. Here is one account:

> The baby I'm taking care of now is a twitty little preemie. She is the ultimate preemie. All you have to do is walk in front of her isolette and have a shadow fall across her face and she desaturates. She cannot stand knowing there is anyone else in the world, but I found that I was able to suction her by myself and keep her saturation in the 90s just by being slow and careful. This baby usually has terrible bradycardia and desaturations when she is suctioned. She developed a reputation for being a real little nerd, but I haven't had any problem with her for the first couple of hours (Tanner, et al. 1993: p. 278).

One might wish to question the interpretation that the baby 'cannot stand knowing there is anyone else in the world' and one might be alarmed by moral judgements revealed by language such as 'nerd'. Nevertheless, I think one has to look beyond such reactions to see the thoughtfulness that has enabled this nurse to take a different approach with this baby, with some initial success. She has not swallowed the judgement that this baby is merely a 'little nerd' and has stepped beyond a collective sense of frustration to take a careful look. Through both observation of the baby and reflection on how this baby makes her feel as its carer, she has come to see the baby differently and the baby has responded. This nurse now knows more about the baby but she also, I would claim, *knows* her a little better than before.

Appropriate privacy

Seen from this perspective, it can perhaps be suggested that a nurse's need to know a lot of facts about a patient on admission, or thereafter, is to some extent defensive against the threat of an encounter with strangers and a reactionary and compensatory extension of power. If we could more easily accept 'not knowing', as neonatal nurses have to do, and used our eyes and our feelings, we might come to know our patients far better than if we feel compelled to invade their psyches with questions. In saying this, of course, I am not meaning to imply that there is never any place for questions; it is finally a matter of balance. However, the more nurses close the space between nurse and patient with preconceived ideas about what sort of relationship should be developing, the less space the nurse is allowing for the patient to form the relationship that he or she wants and possibly needs.

By suggesting that it might be more respectful and more productive to allow patients to determine the nature of the nurse–patient relationship, I am not implying that the patient is at liberty to form any kind of relationship with the nurse, for example, to relate to her as a friend or a potential lover, or turn her into a servant. Any such approaches will be met with a response that conveys to the patient that this is some kind of mistake, that, while it may be understandable, it is not acceptable. As has been previously noted, such boundary drawing protects the privacy of both the patient and the nurse and permits the survival of the professional encounter.

In connection with this, but using a more subtle example, I want to suggest that the nurse has more to do than merely to refrain from unnecessary incursions into the patient's privacy through the asking of questions. She may have a positive duty to help the patient to maintain privacy. The partial intimacy of the nurse–patient relationship may invite a degree of disclosure that the patient subsequently comes to regret. I suggest that nursing could quite properly involve helping a person to anticipate this and thus retain better control of what is shared. One could, therefore, see nursing work that promotes this as expressing respect for the patient's autonomy and as a gesture of the empowerment of patients.

Much current nursing literature is, however, concerned with the reverse problem of how to facilitate rather than help to curtail communication with patients. Mine is not a counterargument; it is rather an attempt to look at the other side of the coin and to suggest that nursing needs to keep hold of both perspectives. An illustration will perhaps make this clearer.

> Moira found the nurse caring for her child to be remarkably warm and caring. One night as they talked of Moira's fears, guilt, and difficulties in coping with her daughter's chronic illness, Moira found herself confiding thoughts and feelings of a very intimate nature in great detail. She cried, laughed, and looked at her plight from all angles, marveling at the ability of this nurse to grasp what she was feeling. Later, as she sat with her daughter through another diagnostic procedure, she began to feel embarrassed about her discussion with the nurse. She realized that she knew virtually nothing personal about the nurse and felt naked and exposed in comparison. She wished that she could take back some of the things she had said and never felt quite as comfortable with the nurse again (Marck, 1990: p. 55).

Marck (1990: p. 56) suggests that the awkwardness might have been resolved by the nurse reciprocating with self-disclosure or by simply thanking the client for sharing such information. This, she says, 'may have been all that was required to "equalize" the client's uncomfortable sense of a one-way giving of personal knowledge, and a one-way taking of listening'.

I do not want to refute these suggestions, but simply to introduce another idea. Perhaps it would have been equally helpful if, at some stage in their conversation, the nurse had noted the closeness between her and this mother and gently reminded her of the reality of the context of their encounter and of its limits. For example, as a nurse she could not be fully the patient's friend and inevitably this made the relationship lopsided. This would have allowed the mother to take stock of what she was saying and to limit it if she wanted to. The intimacy of the dark, the uninterrupted space to talk, may be disinhibiting and, as nurses, we may need to be careful that we are not so charmed and flattered by a person's disclosure of information to us that we fail to see how, from the patient's point of view, the situation is seductive in its invitation to reveal.

Conclusion

I have suggested that if one follows a certain noninstrumental interpretation of what privacy is and why it matters in our lives, this seems to lead to a strong nursing duty to protect it. Refraining from unjustified intrusion is not enough. There may be occasions when nurses need actively to help patients to guard this dimension of themselves, in particular when it comes to the disclosure of information. This idea, if it has any purchase, obviously has to be kept in balance with the importance of receiving disclosures and not leaving patients with a sense of profound isolation. Achieving such a balance clearly requires subtle evaluation.

Acknowledgements

My thanks to my colleagues in the Centre for Philosophy and Health Care (University of Wales, Swansea) for their helpful comments.

References

Altman, I. (1975). *The Environment and Social Behaviour: Privacy, Personal Space, Territory, Crowding.* Brooks/Cole.

Derlega, V.J. and Chaikin, A.L. (1977). Privacy and self-disclosure in social relationships. *J. Soc. Issues*, 33(3), 102–115.

Fried, C. (1984). Privacy: a moral analysis. In *Philosophical Dimensions of Privacy: an Anthology* (F.D. Schoeman, ed.) pp. 203–222, Cambridge University Press.

Girard, M. (1988). Technical expertise as an ethical form: towards an ethics of distance. *J. Med. Ethics*, 14, 25–30.

Marck, P. (1990). Therapeutic reciprocity: a caring phenomenon. *Adv. Nurs. Sci.*, 13(1), 49–59.

May, C. (1992). Nursing work, nurse's knowledge, and the subjectification of the patient. *Sociol. Health Illness*, 14(42), 472–487.

May, C. (1993). Subjectivity and culpability in the constitution of nurse–patient relationships. *Int. J. Nurs. Stud.*, 30(2), 181–192.

May, C. (1995). Patient autonomy and the politics of professional relationships. *J. Adv. Nurs.*, 21, 83–87.

Sacks, O. (1986). *A Leg to Stand On.* Pan.

Salvage, J. (1990). The theory and practice of the new nursing [occasional paper]. *Nurs. Times*, 86(4), 42–45.

Tanner, C.A., Benner, P., Chesla, C. and Gordon, D.R. (1993). The phenomenology of knowing the patient. *Image*, 215, 273–280.

Taylor, B. (1993). 'Ordinariness' in nursing: a study (part I). *Nurs. Stand.*, 7(39), 35–38.

Wellman, C. (1978). A new conception of human rights. In *Human Rights* (E. Kamenka and A.E. Tay, eds) pp. 48–58, Edward Arnold.

Williams, I. (1990). Legal rights and privacy in the information society. In *Law and the State in Modern Times* (W. Maihoffer and G. Sprenger, eds) pp. 218–230, Franz Steiner.

Section Three

Developing the practitioner

Introduction

Diane Wells

This third and final section is concerned with the training and development of psychosocial practitioners.

If we want holistic care, we had better start with whole practitioners; it is not a matter of gaining skills like add-on units. People change whilst working at the Cassel Hospital, and that is how practice can be changed. Psychosocial nursing occurs within a relationship, and that means that feelings are aroused in the practitioner as well as in the client. These feelings are the precious substance which, if examined carefully, can inform the practitioner of the work to be undertaken.

The authors in this section describe how they help nurses to develop skills of working with relationships; the last two, in particular, give personal accounts of how they themselves learned whilst at the Cassel Hospital. A central aspect of this learning work is small discussion groups known as Balint-style seminars. Michael Balint, a psychoanalyst, developed this kind of seminar work with general practitioners at the Tavistock Clinic in the 1950s. He emphasized the role of the seminar leader as one of engendering a spirit of enquiry, respecting the practitioner's attempt to help the patient, and keeping the practitioner–patient relationship as the focus of study. Psychoanalytical theory emphasizes the importance of examining the emotions aroused in the practitioner by the patient. The aim is to help practitioners to make their own discoveries for themselves, rather than telling them about theories, or what to do.

Doreen Clifford, mentor to many authors in this volume, writes about her work in Balint-style psychosexual seminars. She explains how a seminar provides the practitioner with a model of what it is like to be listened to and understood. Meanings are unravelled, and defences are gently questioned, so that nurses can perceive the distress that is often latent in a patient's question, such as: 'Is it all right?' Then, a nurse may be able to transfer what has been experienced in the seminar and face the pain with the patient. Solutions, or comfort, are not inevitable consequences, but they can be achieved when distress is recognized.

'How can I help?' is about Charlie McGrory's attempts to help general nursing students to understand their experiences with mentally ill patients. The students' minds were focused on exams, and for much of the time they seemed unable to think about their relationships with patients. However, in one seminar there was a major breakthrough, and some students were able to understand the parallel between being heard in the seminar and hearing the distress of a patient, instead of merely offering reassurance.

In 'Biographical work with older people', I give examples to show how nurses develop psychosocial aspects of care with older people. This work is supported not only with Balint-style seminars but also with literature on social gerontology, which promotes a biographical approach to understanding later life. When I returned to discuss these examples with the practitioners, months later, I heard how difficult it is to sustain the work; the culture of care often sets limits on the practitioner's interpretation of individualized care.

Mic Rafferty describes how clinical supervision can provide practitioners with the support and learning opportunities they need in order to be truly accountable for their practice. He uses examples from his programmes on clinical supervision to show the importance of an environment in which practitioners can feel held in order that they can, in turn, hold the anxieties of their patients and, sometimes, their colleagues. The course provides opportunities to explore the reasons for actions and their effects, and, most importantly, opportunities to monitor the giving of self. Here, supervision is a self-imposed and mutually negotiated scrutiny, which helps the nurse to achieve accountability and maintain sensitivity, with minimal damage to patient and practitioner.

Sonia Stephen describes vividly, from an Afrocentric perspective, what she learned from her five years as a nurse at the Cassel Hospital. While there, she was 'Miss English', fully integrated into the hospital culture, which reflected the society outside in that race was not on the agenda.

Although there was an attempt to understand class, gender and group dynamics, the social order went largely unchallenged. However, she learned something extremely valuable: to articulate what she saw and what she felt. These abilities were used not only to help patients but also to analyse her own position. This was a seed for change.

Louise de Lambert gives a personal account of her first weeks at the Cassel Hospital. She captures the intensity of the experience, when learning is achieved by reflecting on the feelings aroused on working with patients and colleagues. Louise gives examples to show how she has used this approach when leading Balint-style seminars. She argues that practitioners develop their skills when feelings are respected. The powerful feelings described, the need to monitor the giving of self, and the constraints often placed on relationship work with patients, suggest that individualized care requires emotionally skilled practitioners, and is a radical departure from traditions in caring work.

Chapter 11
Psychosexual nursing seminars

Doreen Clifford

This chapter describes how, in a supportive group of colleagues, shared reflective practice can enhance nurses' skills in responding to the psychosexual problems of their patients. Examples from a variety of settings are used to show something of the differing needs of patients, and how seminar work can provide clinical supervision, professional development and support to nurses.

Nurses are continually being met by patients' requests (often disguised) for help with their sexual worries, particularly at times of strain, pain and change in their lives. For example, following surgery, childbirth, bereavement or a renewal of sexual activity. Masked as it may be by other difficulties, such as loss of a breast or cancer, it is easy to overlook and avoid psychosexual pain. The problem may be reinforced by the nurse's shyness and reluctance to take risks in such a sensitive area. It is no wonder that some patients haunt general practitioners' surgeries, family planning clinics and other places, seeking relief for the unspeakable distress that neither they nor we understand. We have all met them and been puzzled and irritated by them, but perhaps have failed to understand and address their difficulties. Sexuality may seem frivolous in the face of illness, mutilation or approaching death, except to the person concerned. For example, a woman in her mid-thirties, newly widowed, was diagnosed with cancer of the bladder. She begged the surgeon not to remove her uterus along with the bladder, but no enquiry was made about why this was so important to her. During subsequent years of treatment, no one ever asked her about her sexuality, her wishes, fears or needs.

Psychosexual seminar training with experienced nurses

Today, there is increasing recognition that nurses in training and in practice need to develop skills of reflection on their work with patients. The seminar method is a tried and tested technique of experiential learning, using shared reflection in groups of professional health care-workers. These techniques were first evolved by Michael and Enid Balint in their work with general practitioners, and further developed by Tom Main in his work with family planning doctors (later to become the Institute of Psychosexual Medicine) (Balint, 1957; Main, 1989). Such Balint-type seminars are a central aspect of psychosocial nurse training and support at the Cassel Hospital, and provide a model for working with specifically psychosexual issues.

A psychosexual nursing seminar is composed of six to ten post-registration nurses engaged in similar kinds of work. The aim is to reflect on their day-to-day work in order to improve their skills in responding sensitively to patients. Members are invited to describe their encounters with patients who have presented with sexual health care needs, especially those that left the nurses feeling uneasy or dissatisfied with the response they offered. The task of the group is to listen carefully to the nurse's description of an encounter, and to explore the nature of the nurse–patient relationship. For example, why did *this* nurse go out of her way to please *this* patient, only to find herself feeling useless and inadequate?

The group gives each nurse support and space for reflection, the opportunity to develop fresh skills, and confidence to discuss sexual issues with patients where appropriate. When the seminar is working well, it provides for each member a model of what it is like to be listened to and understood, and an experience of working together in exploring the complexity of the feelings expressed in the nurse–patient encounter. Alexis Brook (1980) describes 'the experience of feeling understood' as a central process of counselling. Nurses, similarly, can find that a supportive seminar group provides a place in which they can feel understood by their colleagues. At no time, however, is a seminar group used for personal counselling or group therapy. Nurses who feel understood are more able to provide their patients with this understanding, although the responsibility for feelings and action remains always with the patient.

Some examples of nursing work brought to seminars

A midwife, new to the seminar, reported visiting a postnatal patient at home. On each of four visits the mother asked if 'down below' was all right. The midwife looked at a nicely healing perineum and said all was well on each occasion. Only after they had said goodbye did the midwife wonder whether she had missed an opportunity to explore what lay behind the patient's questions. On discussing this in the seminar, she realized that she had avoided responding to the patient's request for a chance to talk over her anxieties following childbirth.

Even experienced nurses are often faced with the problem of timing. When would be the best moment to start talking about sexual issues with patients? The fear of rejection at speaking too soon must be balanced against the risk of losing the opportunity by waiting too long. The ability to raise such issues, however, can give patients the opportunity to discuss worries which they might otherwise find difficult to speak about.

For example, a general practice nurse described a smartly dressed older woman who came because she thought she needed a smear test. 'You look very well,' said the nurse, bustling about in preparation. 'We've just returned from Paris, the first time my husband and I have been there together.' 'Did you have a good time?' asked the nurse. She found this sophisticated woman formidable but dared to ask: 'How was your lovemaking?' 'Well that's why I've come, really. It was wonderful. Is that all right at my age? I'm over 70, you see and we haven't had intercourse for some years.' After she had talked this through with the nurse, she decided that she did not require a smear test after all and left, apparently satisfied.

Why had this woman come to see the nurse? Was she perhaps seeking reassurance that the pleasure and excitement of her sexuality were still acceptable? The response that she received from the nurse seemed to enable her to ask the real questions that she needed to address, and the physical examination was not required.

Sometimes, the nurse–patient encounter can provide information about the patient's relationship with a spouse or partner. For example, a nurse reported to the seminar how understanding she had been in helping a patient to avoid a vaginal examination about which she (the patient) was very anxious. During the seminar discussion, the nurse came to recognize that she had colluded with the patient in avoiding the issue of her anxiety about being examined. The next time they met in the clinic, the nurse commented: 'I noticed you were reluctant to have that examination last time. Do you have some difficulties with this?' The patient smiled: 'Oh yes nurse, I have problems with intercourse but my husband is very kind, he doesn't insist.' When the nurse discussed this further in the seminar group, it became clearer that she had colluded with the defences used so skilfully by this patient to avoid the difficulties in her sexual life. The nurse realized that, like the husband, she had avoided discussing the wife's evasion of entry to her vagina, thus perhaps confirming the patient's fear that her problem was hopeless. Through her work in the seminar, the nurse began to formulate a more appropriate response to this patient.

The problem of involvement

Most of us enter the nursing profession because we want to do something about suffering, yet our training often helps us to build defences against recognizing suffering in others. In some instances, technical competence actually depends on our suppressing our normal human reactions, in the operating theatre or intensive care unit, for instance. The uncomfortable work of studying one's own feelings in relation to patients is something that nurse training usually avoids. When we defend ourselves against the pain of not knowing what to do, by reassurance, giving good advice, perhaps, or unthinkingly referring-on, we can fail to address our patients' real needs. When the painful feelings evoked in the nurse are identified and understood in the seminar, that understanding becomes the basis for continuing work with the patient.

In a seminar, fears of 'getting too involved' with patients are challenged. As nurses, we have no choice *but* to be involved. To deny involvement is to negate the patient's need to be understood. To become overinvolved is to risk being useless. Involvement supported by professional self-reflection, however, can give us the means to stay with the pain evoked in us by our patients, rather than defend ourselves against it. Human pain and suffering require a response that goes beyond the practical issues of physical care. The capacity to reflect on our own reactions to patients can provide us with a vital tool for understanding and responding to their distress, as can be seen from the next example.

The bikers' story

The nurse was the last one in the family planning clinic that evening, as the receptionist had been called away early. Only one more patient to see: 'Next!' Two huge bikers, clad in black leather from head to foot, loomed over her. She was momentarily terrified. 'How can I help you?' They sat down and held hands. 'I'm a failure,' he said with tears in his eyes. 'Can't satisfy her. It won't stay up. I love her so much and let her down all the time.' The girl hugged him. 'It really doesn't matter,' she said to the nurse, who responded by saying: 'Tell me.'

They had fallen madly in love, and had been together a year, but he could never maintain an erection. 'It has taken us months to get here. We were so afraid someone would laugh.'

The nurse took their medical history but could think of nothing useful to say and felt utterly hopeless. Finally, she offered to see the young man alone the following week. He was pleased. 'No promises,' she said.

The nurse had recently joined a psychosexual seminar, and this was her first case to report. 'Tell me what to do!' she pleaded with the group. They helped the nurse to reflect on the feelings she had brought to the seminar: terror, compassion, liking, anxiety, hopelessness and despair. They helped her to understand that her hopelessness was a reflection of the young man's feelings. They recognized her skill at enabling the couple to show their pain of repeated failure. Could the nurse keep her head, stop to think about her feelings, and try to see to whom they belonged when next she met the young man?

He came in alone. The girl waited for him outside as he told the same story of continuing failure. Again the nurse felt a terrible hopelessness, but this time, realized that the hopelessness was his, and not hers. She asked, 'Can you remember how it felt when you first failed to get an erection?' He sat quietly. 'I'd forgotten. Haven't thought of it for years.' In mounting distress, he told of being seduced at the age of 16 by a friend of his mother's who took him to bed and then laughed at his small penis when he failed to get an erection. The nurse was very moved but contained her feelings and asked: 'How did that make you feel?' Now came his anger and rage about how this experience had robbed him of his potency and his feelings of manhood for all these years.

In this case, the nurse had bravely recognized her own feelings, reflected on them with colleagues, and used them to guide her response to the young man's distress. This response allowed him, in his turn, to recognize the feelings which lay behind his sexual impotence.

Working with feelings

Developing the ability to work with feelings and 'think on one's feet' is not easy. Most of us are too well trained in wanting to *do* something, get on, get finished, make it better. This is where psychosexual nursing seminars offer continuing training whilst providing the best professional supervision and support system we have.

Feelings do not just go away. Unresolved distress can emerge in apparently unrelated symptoms, such as depression, headaches and general ill health, and may provoke unexplained absences. Seminar groups can be powerful forums for learning. Listening closely to the reflections on each other's work puts members in touch with the feelings experienced at the time of the encounter with the patient. We can check these feelings with each other by asking for more information about what was experienced at the time, or what was understood on reflection. Because the disturbance of experiencing another's distress is the daily work of all seminar members, they are quick to recognize such feelings in each other. This gives the opportunity for that spark of recognition, of having been there oneself. Thus, an open and honest description of what actually occurred in the nurse–patient relationship can be presented. This provides an atmosphere of trust, where criticism, whatever the material presented, is suspended. Criticism in the group, when it occurs, usually reflects some aspect of the nurse–patient relationship.

A psychosexual problem after mastectomy

The next example shows that when group members feel a sense of unease about an encounter, although the presenting nurse's story is of a perfectly ordinary meeting, it may reveal something about what happened for the nurse. The nurse can then use these new understandings in the next meeting with that patient.

The prosthesis nurse was visiting a postoperative mastectomy patient. As part of the conversation, she enquired about the husband's feelings. The patient became visibly upset. The nurse reassured her and quickly left. Subsequently, she had phone calls from the patient enquiring about further appointments to fit the prosthesis.

There was a rich discussion when this was reported to the seminar. It covered the patient's grief at the loss of her breast, her fear of death associated with cancer, and her need for comfort and reassurance, as shown by the telephone calls. The group members reassured the nurse about the quality of her work. The leader, however, pointed out that it was when the nurse mentioned the husband that the patient's distress had become apparent. Was there something more here? The seminar group then addressed the possibility of unexplored anxiety about the patient's sexual life and wondered what lay behind the repeated telephone calls.

The presenting nurse found these ideas threatening and was reluctant to discuss sex as a likely difficulty for the patient. The leader showed the group how their reassurance of the nurse had echoed the nurse's reassurance of the patient; on each occasion the trigger to distress had been ignored. The nurse was also reflecting the patient's reluctance to explore the sexual implications of the mastectomy. That the patient had hope in and trusted the nurse was, however, evident from the phone calls.

At the following meeting, the nurse reported how, for the first time ever, at the prosthesis fitting she had shyly asked if lovemaking was all right. The patient wept, said she had not spoken about the loss of her breast to her husband, and told how she had repulsed his affectionate advances. The nurse and the patient shared the sadness of this situation. Later, another phone call followed. The patient had talked to her husband of her feelings. They had cried together then 'one thing led to another and it's all right now, thanks'. There was general delight in the group, and the leader pointed out how the nurse's act of understanding and sharing with the patient had been later mirrored in the husband–wife relationship.

Some training outcomes

The outcomes from seminar training are as varied as the nurses taking part. One midwife now sees the postnatal visit as a place where it is appropriate to ask: 'How is lovemaking for you after the baby?' and to be ready to discuss the response. Some family planning nurses have felt it their responsibility to set aside time before or after normal clinic sessions to see patients in difficulty. They often give their own time for this. Another midwife, feeling that antenatal clinics were formidable places for people to ask questions freely, approached a mother and baby shop for space where once a week she held a stall labelled YOUR QUESTIONS ANSWERED. She had a multitude of people approaching her on topics ranging from sadness following the death of a baby to what kind of nappies to buy. The shop enjoyed the extra custom.

The majority of seminar-trained nurses remain in their chosen specialty, continuing with their ordinary work but with a heightened response to patients' psychosexual health care needs. Some go on for further training and a few move into counselling. A number of experienced nurses have been appointed as nurse specialists in psychosexual counselling.

The development of psychosexual nurse training

In 1973, in response to nurses' requests for training to help them to deal with patients who were presenting with psychosexual problems, the Family Planning Association with the Department of Health initiated research into the appropriateness of psychosexual seminar training for family planning nurses. Using findings from the seminar leaders' research, the Joint Board of Clinical Nursing Studies set up what was to become ENB 985 Principles of Psychosexual Counselling for Nurses (Selby, 1985; Randall, 1992).

From these beginnings in family planning, nurses in many specialties have grown to recognize that patients' sexual health care needs are an integral part of their nursing task. Whether hospital nurses, physiotherapists, nurses from Stoke Mandeville Hospital for spinal injuries, midwives, health visitors, or nurses working in general practice, family planning, continence care with children and the elderly, and oncology, all have sought help to develop skills in responding appropriately to the sexual health care needs of patients. Many nurses are still seeking help to develop these skills.

Since 1980, a small group of nurse seminar leaders have responded to this need by running brief workshops and regular seminars across the UK. This work has provided a rich source of data about nurses' difficulties in responding to patients' requests for help. Some common explanations for these difficulties were:

- Lack of time
- Not enough knowledge
- Too embarrassed
- Fear of giving wrong advice
- Personal inexperience
- Lack of confidence
- Not enough privacy
- Personal inadequacy

These reasons can be seen as nurses expressing their (perceived) inadequacy in responding to patients' needs. It is clear that for some nurses this is an easy and ordinary part of their working lives, but the majority find it a cause for anxiety and denial, even when the patient's needs are openly expressed.

Another finding was the defensiveness many nurses develop in order to avoid the painful work of recognizing and responding to patients in need of help with their psychosexual distress. Nurses, in turn, require help to discuss and understand this defensiveness and its roots in their previous experience, including their training.

Gaining recognition for psychosexual nursing

It is noteworthy that doctors have for some time been able to obtain the recognition of psychosexual skills under the auspices of the Institute of Psychosexual Medicine. There is a Diploma in Sexual Health Care, which is a multidisciplinary training using behaviourist methods, held at one of the teaching hospitals. There has been no similar recognition for psychosexual seminar-trained nurses.

By the time people read this book, however, there will be an Association of Psychosexual Nurses working towards gaining university accreditation for psychosexual seminar training. This association derives from a countrywide Psychosexual Nursing Network which has met twice-yearly for study days in London since 1986. Speakers have included a nurse who helped to develop family planning services in Romania, a nurse working with the Bangladeshi community in East London, another reporting on an experiment in sex education in a South London school, and a nurse specialist describing her experiences with infertility work.

There are already a number of basic psychosexual nursing seminars running in London and Maidstone, and continuing seminars in London, Bristol, Ipswich and Winchester. Basic introductory seminar groups meet regularly every two weeks, for six terms of six seminars, over two years. Similarly, continuation seminars meet fortnightly. In London there is an advanced seminar for psychosexual nurse counsellors and also a seminar for nurse seminar leaders. An experienced psychosexual nurse leader in Bristol has set up workshops and seminars for nurse tutors to develop ways of integrating psychosexual understanding into the general nursing curriculum. The work of psychosexual nurse training continues to develop.

The costs of this training, in time and commitment, need to be set alongside the quality of nursing care that results (Randall, 1992). An immediate nursing response to psychosexual distress can save hours of time and treatment by a multiplicity of other health care workers, and years of hidden human misery. The profit and loss of financial resources set aside for such training need to be considered in the light of such findings.

Psychosexual seminar training does not require a leader who is an expert in sexual dysfunction. It requires someone who is trained and practised in paying attention to the reactions of the group, to the reporting nurse, and to the study of the nurse–patient relationship. Such seminar training is, however, lengthy. Fresh thinking requires time if it is to be installed into the mind. Knowledge that has been gained previously over a long period is not readily set aside for newly-met ideas and practice, however rewarding (Main, 1967). Under the stress of not knowing how to respond to a particular difficulty, and without appropriate support, it can be easier to regress to 'knowing best', which requires less thought and effort.

As well as seminars for trained nurses, there is also a need for tutorial training for student nurses. The area of patients' sexual health care is beginning to be addressed in text books and training courses, but the subject of students' feelings generally remains neglected. Even now, nurses are seldom enabled in their basic training to see that psychosexual work is a necessary part of their professional response to patients. Many, therefore, feel that their natural feelings of awkwardness and shyness in this area are wrong and should not be spoken about. Although, as students, nurses are taught to care intimately for seriously ill men and women, frequently washing and handling breasts and genitalia, they are seldom given any help with the feelings this might arouse in them or their patients. An opportunity for students to reflect upon and discuss such feelings, in small tutorial groups, could form the basis for recognizing the implications of such feelings for them and their patients. They could be encouraged to appreciate when these feelings are likely to occur, and develop their nursing skills in, for instance, recognizing the needs of patients for privacy and sensitivity in daily care. Such tutorials would also give an opportunity for tutors to be alert to the strain their students might be undergoing, which, in turn, could set a model for the students of recognizing, valuing and responding to patients' experiences.

Psychosexual nursing skills need to be developed through seminar training as an integral part of both pre- and postgraduate training. Such training and support will improve nurses' ability to respond skilfully to spoken and unspoken requests for help with the human suffering they meet in their everyday work.

References

Balint, M. (1957). *The Doctor, His Patient and the Illness*. Pitman Medical.
Brook, A. (1980). Brief psychotherapy in clinical practice. *Medicine* 3rd series, **36**, 1834–1836.
Main, T.F. (1967). Knowledge, learning and freedom from thought. *Aust. N. Z. J. Psychiatry*, **1**, 64–71
Main, T.F. (J. Johns, ed.) (1989). *The Ailment and other Psychoanalytic Essays*. Free Association Books.
Randall, E. (1992). *Preparation for Psychosexual Nursing*. The Centre for Inner City Studies, Goldsmith's College.
Selby, J. (1985). Close encounters. *Nurs. Times*, **78**(17), 8.

Further reading

Balint, E. and Norel, J.S., eds. (1973). *Six Minutes for the Patient*. Tavistock Publications.
Barnes, E., ed. (1968). *Psychosocial Nursing: Studies from the Cassel Hospital*. Tavistock Publications.
Brook, A. (1983). A psychotherapeutic approach in medical practice. *Med. Int.*, **34**, 1618–1620.
Casement, P. (1985). *On Learning from the Patient*. Tavistock Publications.
Cole, B. (1993). *Mummy Laid an Egg!* Jonathan Cape.
Endacott, J. (1989). Coping with psychosexual problems. *Nurs. Stand.*, **3**(42).
Menzies, I.E.P. (1976). *The Functioning of Social Systems as a Defence Against Anxiety*. Tavistock Publications.
Selby, J. (1989). Psychosexual nursing. In *Introduction to Psychosexual Medicine* (R. Skrine, ed.) pp. 134–147, Chapman and Hall.
Selby, J. (1990). Psychosexual nursing. *Pract. Nurse*, **3**(2), 99–101.
Tunnadine, P. (1979). *Contraception and Sexual Life*. Institute of Psychosexual Medicine.
Tunnadine, P. (1993). Training groups in psychosexual medicine. *Int. J. Ther. Communities*, **14**(4), 257–264.

Chapter 12
How can I help?

Charlie McGrory

This chapter draws upon research work undertaken as part of degree studies, which attempted to identify a role for the nurse teacher in the clinical setting. The basis for the research was work undertaken with adult nursing students on a traditional, certificate-level course during their mental health placement. It was hoped that a role could be identified which would indicate how a teacher might influence, positively, the students' views of mentally ill individuals and how they could be cared for. The core of the work was expressed more directly by a student's questioning; 'How can I help?' On looking back, this appears to be a clearer expression of the issues involved in attempting to identify a role, while struggling with the changes taking place in nurse education and practice. The issues to be discussed include: the mental health placement; the theory–practice gap; educationalists as clinical teachers; and aspects of my research with the students relating to their mental health placements, in particular, their dealing with distress in face-to-face encounters with patients.

Although the research focused on the mental health placement for adult nursing, the issues it raised are of relevance to the education and practice of nurses in other settings.

Mental health placements

In England and Wales, a placement in a mental health setting has been a requirement of the education of general nurses since 1977 (General

Nursing Council, 1977). The overall aim of such placements is for students to gain knowledge and skills in recognizing mental illness and promoting mental health. However, research studies indicate that the mental health placement has little effect upon students' attitudes toward the mentally ill. Studies note that students' attitudes prior to the placement include feelings of apprehension, anxiety and fearfulness toward psychiatric patients. At the end of the placements, the overall attitude change had been minimal. Students remained fearful (Wilkinson, 1982) and anxious (Scott, 1990; Procter and Haffner, 1991), and, after four months, any positive changes were reversed after the students returned to general nursing (Collister, 1983).

Theory–practice gap and clinical teaching

The failure of my discussion groups to change the attitudes of these nurses can be seen as another example of the widely accepted 'theory–practice' gap in nurse education (Bendall, 1975; Hawkett, 1990; McCaugherty, 1991a; Nolan and Grant 1992). The educationalists' aims that students should gain knowledge and skills in the field of mental illness are not borne out in practice.

Clinical teaching by educationalists has been proposed to mitigate the theory–practice gap. However, the literature on this subject indicates that clinical teachers and nurse tutors (Jones, 1985) are unable to carry out clinical teaching because of classroom teaching commitments, role-strain difficulties, and problems in establishing a credible clinical presence. In reviewing the changing role of the nurse teacher, Crotty and Butterworth (1992) and Crotty (1993) note the minimal time devoted to clinical teaching and the rejection of a role involving direct care of patients. Gerrish (1992) questions the effect of attempting to remedy these issues by establishing one grade of teacher to be responsible for all aspects of nurse education. Given these problems, it is not surprising that exhortations (Webster, 1990) for teachers to share in their students 'messy, indeterminate real practice situations' (Greenwood, 1993) have had little impact.

Adult learning and experiential learning

The work of Knowles (1980) on adult learners and learning has become popular in nurse education (Quinn, 1988; Burnard, 1989). Adult learning emphasizes the recognition of learners as adults with a wealth of experience, seeking relevance, and wishing to be active, rather than passive, in the process of learning. This approach has undeniable intrinsic attractiveness and potential value in nurse education. However, its adoption in nurse education seems to overlook its theoretical and philosophical underpinning and its background origins, which arise in the student-centred work of Rogers (Kirschenbaum and Henderson, 1990).

Individual adults are assumed to be rational in behaviour, or moving toward rationality. Insufficient attention is directed towards anxiety arising from psychic conflicts (Hinshelwood, 1987). The conflicts arise from the intimacy of contact in the relationship between nurse and patient, which mobilizes defences to ward off primitive libidinal and aggressive impulses (Menzies, 1970). In her study of general nursing students, Menzies described the defences employed by nursing as a group and nurses as individuals. Some of the defences include the use of task organization, which splits the nurse–patient relationship into a series of separate tasks, delegating decision making to superiors to reduce full responsibility, and the use of projection. Such defences indicate how mistaken it may be to assume that behaviour is governed by rationality.

Experiential learning attempts to address the issue of learning arising from direct experience, although its value may be limited by the use of defences. Burnard (1989) suggests that experiential learning may support the development of experiential knowledge derived through direct encounters with people and situations. For learning to take place, a necessary structure is required, which takes account of the defences. Without this, it is probable that difficulties arising from defending against anxiety (Menzies, 1970) may overwhelm individuals and prevent learning taking place. Boydell (1976) suggests an experiential learning cycle, which may provide such a structure; this is shown in Figure 12.1.

Students are encouraged to identify and discuss problems and perceptions, to examine cognition, affect and conation (behaviour), and to derive actions for future applications. The process relies on the creation of an environment where individuals can reflect on the problems with which they are engaged. This process leads to a consideration of reflective practice popularized by the works from America of Schön (1983, 1987, 1991) and taken up avidly, as illustrated by British literature (Powell, 1989; Jarvis, 1992; McCaugherty, 1991b; Atkins and Murphy, 1993; Coutts-Jarman, 1993; Greenwood, 1993; Reed and Procter, 1993; Reid, 1993). The list is not exhaustive, merely illustrative of what may be considered a current preoccupation in nurse education or, possibly, a current fad.

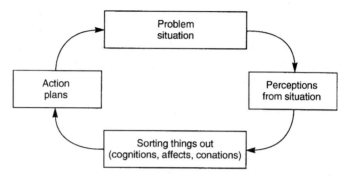

Figure 12.1   Experiential learning cycle (after Boydell, 1976).

To regard Schön's work as a quickly passing fad would be to fail to recognize the value of the dichotomy depicted in the statement: 'In the varied topography of professional practice there is a high, hard ground overlooking a swamp' (Schön, 1987: p. 3). In the realm of the high ground, problems are solved by applying research-based theory and technique, while in swampy lowlands, problems of practice refuse to be solved by technical rationality. A swampy lowland for nurses and other health professionals is in the nature of interpersonal relationships with patients. However, Schön's work on reflection is often discussed in terms of reflection-on-action, or reflection-in-action, and this can result in a focus upon the action, or rather activity, of motor skills, which is right and proper but neglects the domain of interpersonal relationships which are problematic for nurses.

A central feature of nurse training at the Cassel Hospital has been a Balint-style seminar (Balint, 1957), convened to provide nurses with the opportunity of investigating the interpersonal relationships with patients. Inevitably, the relationships discussed are predominantly those that puzzle, worry and in some way threaten the capacity of highly motivated and experienced nurses to provide care for patients.

The seminar approach recognizes that engaging with patients may mobilize defences against the often painful experiences that such contacts bring. An arena is provided (a 'practicum' in Schön's terms) in which issues from there and then can be explored in the here and now with the aim of allowing defensive manoeuvres to be identified, and to some extent, modified. In her work, Menzies (1970) identifies the range of defences nurses use as individuals and as a body to help to cope with the anxiety that arises in everyday work. It seemed to be possible that this seminar approach may be of value in helping student nurses to investigate the experience of the mental health placement in which they find themselves, and to contribute to the development of a more positive attitude toward mental illness.

Research method

The frequency of student groups undertaking placement allowed the possibility for comparing the outcome on student attitudes when a Balint-style seminar was provided for one group of students but not for another.

The method developed for enquiring into the value of the seminar approach was to measure the students' attitudes before and after the placement of two groups of general nurse students. One group (A) was offered the opportunity to meet a nurse teacher on ten occasions throughout the mental health placement at a predetermined time, at a location on one of the wards where the students worked. For both groups, progress in the placement was monitored by visits to the ward areas and discussions with nurse managers and mentors. However, group B did not have formal meetings with a nurse teacher to discuss their experiences. The attitude measures used were those devised by Wilkinson (1982), using repertory grid technique to analyse students' responses to 12 clinical vignettes depicting six medical histories and six psychiatric histories. Both groups were approaching the end of their second year of training and had similar clinical placements. One individual had previous experience of caring for the mentally ill when employed as a nursing assistant. The general characteristics of the groups are shown in Table 12.1.

The aims of the discussions for group A were explained to the group by the researcher when enlisting their participation in the research and again at the initial meeting:

> The meeting is intended to offer you an opportunity to discuss your thoughts and feelings about patients, issues, events and happenings that take place during your mental health placement . . . It is not my intention as a lecturer to come with a predetermined subject either to discuss or teach. Rather I will attempt to participate in discussions in a helpful manner.

Group A comprised 14 student nurses and meetings were arranged on ten occasions. Attendance at the group varied widely. Theoretically, there

Table 12.1 Group characteristics

	Group A (n = 14)	Group B (n = 18)
Age (years)		
Range	21–32	20–33
Mean	25.1	28.5
Standard deviation	4.2	3.8
Gender		
Female	14	16
Male	0	2
Previous experience	0	1

were 140 possible attendances; absences (sickness or off-duty) reduced this to a possible 93, and, finally, only 78 actual attendances were made. This appears comparable with the discussion groups reported by Fabricius (1991). The range of students' attendance was large, between two and nine. It may have been significant that half of the actual attendances were accounted for by five of the 14 students.

Themes from the ten group discussions were placed into six categories using methods of content analysis suggested by the work of Melia (1987) and Burnard (1991). Categories of discussion were identified by reading the records of the discussion group and identifying progressively more inclusive categories into which the items discussed would fit. In this way it was hoped that suggestions for further enquiry and investigation would arise. The six categories identified were:

1. *Study and working:* the students' descriptions and views of the importance and availability of support from clinical and educational staff in preparing for an unseen written examination, which would determine whether the students could continue on their course.
2. *Working on the wards:* the nature of work seen and done by students and the physical environment.
3. *Perception of others:* the students' views of the patients and staff with whom they were in contact.
4. *Responses of students:* describing and talking about their feelings, thoughts and behaviour during the clinical placement.
5. *Perception of own abilities:* students' descriptions of their difficulties in knowing how to respond to patients.
6. *Teacher interventions:* the contributions of the teacher during the discussion groups.

Group discussion

The first theme dominated the first five discussions because, despite further clinical and theoretical assessments, this was the last formal written examination of the students' course and was referred to by students as their 'finals'. Despite the course having a further year to run, the perception of 'finals' by the students caused them high levels of anxiety. They correctly viewed the examination as relating to the theory and practice of general nursing, not to mental illness. Listening to the students repeatedly question the relevance of the mental health placement at this time in their course led eventually to a 'blinding flash of the obvious' quoted from Bion by Dartington (1993).

For a variety of understandable reasons, the examination on physical illness was scheduled during the placement focused on mental illness. The discussion group had been conceived and intended by the researcher to take advantage of the adult learning, experiential and reflective approaches in relation to the placement, but he had singularly failed to put it in the context of the whole curriculum experienced by the students. The relevant learning in which these students wished to be engaged was preparation to pass an examination which was essential to their continued education to become general nurses. Notably, while the students' discussion was dominated by the examination, there were discussions that indicated some evidence of conflict experienced by the students. This was clearly expressed in one student's comment: 'I am interested in mental illness but I will only really think about it and get involved when I know I have passed the exam.'

Discussion dynamics

At the sixth meeting of the discussion group, four students were present: Joanne, Caroline, Susan and Janet. This was the first meeting after the examination. The discussion had opened with Caroline describing a conversation between herself and a student on a course leading to a degree in nursing. They had spoken about Caroline's worry and concern regarding the outcome of the examination taken by the students in this group in the previous week. The nursing degree student had appeared to dismiss her worries, saying it was only a certificate level course and not very hard. It was easy. Caroline was clearly annoyed and other members of the group responded with angry comments. Discussion continued with comparisons between the students' own course and other forms of nurse education.

At this time, nurse education was undergoing a major transition from traditional certificate-level courses to diploma and degree courses. The students were well aware they were on one of the last of the traditional courses and had referred in other meetings to thinking they were now leftovers while nurse teachers concentrated on newer courses at diploma and degree level. There was a sense of vulnerability and questioning of their training, especially about their future careers, with fears that they would be at a disadvantage in comparison with nurses who had diploma or degree qualifications.

The focus of the students' talk became a sharing of the practical skills they possessed and a valuing of how these had helped physically ill patients. Joanne was looking forward to working on Ward 'X' in the future because of the demands for physical care. I felt excluded and, perhaps identifying with other teachers, asked if providing physical care was satisfying because it provided a clearly defined and immediate role, which seemed absent from the students' experience of working in psychiatric wards.

A new input to discussion

Joanne then began to tell us about a patient, Chris, a young man of 19 years. She described a very anxious young man who seemed to have become isolated and alone because he believed he had razor blades on his legs, which would cut people if he got close to them. Joanne said that Chris had been seen on the ward round and had been 'reassured' that he would not hurt people. Chris' mother visited him frequently and also tried to reassure her son that he would not harm people. The reassurance also included telling Chris that he did not have razor blades on his legs. Joanne conveyed a feeling of concern for Chris, coupled with a sense of helplessness. She did not know how to help him. The reassurance, Joanne said, had not diminished the anxiety or the beliefs Chris held. Although Joanne wanted to help Chris, she could not think of how to approach him or what to say, and now consciously avoided him, to escape from her own feeling of discomfort because of her sense of being powerless. Susan now quickly recounted her own avoidance of a young woman on her ward because of similar circumstances. Caroline and Janet said they had also had similar experiences.

This was a marked contrast from the previous discussion about the satisfaction gained from nursing the physically ill. It indicated, I thought, something about feeling vulnerable. In trying to counter my own feeling of helplessness, I asked if the students could think of ways to respond to Chris. Joanne replied forcefully: 'There's too little time left, we can't be experts.' I agreed there was little time left of the placement, and Joanne could not be an expert, but wondered if it was possible to find ways of responding, other than to avoid patients like Chris or the others they had described. Joanne replied vehemently and directly: 'How, how can I help?'

I felt put on the spot and very uncomfortable, perhaps this was just what the students experienced when they were with patients. I was afraid that any reply I made would be disdainfully rejected as theory from a teacher unconnected to the everyday experience of work on a ward. Feeling defensive, I said I was generalizing, but wondered what would happen if they thought about the patient's experience of being alone and frightened; in Chris' case, whether he felt both frightened and frightening. I was aware, however, of the dilemma faced by staff and students of believing that attention to evidently delusional thoughts (which razors on legs appeared to be) encourages and reinforces their existence. The commonly held stance is to ignore such statements, find a means of distracting the patient and, of course, provide some form of reassurance.

However, it is possible that the outcome of such responses may lead to the isolation of the individual patient. In this instance, Chris appears to have been left alone with his alarming perceptions of his situation, as staff and students avoided contact with him and so the discomfort of feeling powerless when reassurance fails to help. The avoidance can be seen, in part, as defending against the distress raised by feeling powerless. However, while Chris may have become isolated, it also appears that students became isolated themselves with their feelings of powerlessness, and this increased the need for defensive actions.

Caroline's next comment seemed to reinforce the need for such defences: 'The razors are only imagination, they aren't really there Why worry about them?' I tried to link Caroline's comment to the earlier discussion of worries and anxieties about the examination by asking if they were only imaginary, and asking also if thinking about feeling might create a sense of being listened to in place of being 'reassured' that it is only a certificate level course and 'it's easy'. It was hoped that this intervention would enable students to focus on their responses when their anxieties went unrecognized and were met with reassurance. If this could

be discussed, it might reduce isolation and allow alternative con-
ceptualizations of both Chris' and their own situations to be considered.

The intervention seemed to have had some effect, because Caroline
then quickly described in detail a personal experience of not being listened
to in a social setting. It had left her with mixed feelings of being alone and
furious because she thought she was being ignored. Joanne then said she
could understand feeling furious and wondered if this was connected to
her avoiding Chris. She had only been able to think of telling Chris he
would not hurt anyone and thought this would not have helped him. It
seemed that Joanne's personal experience of being ignored involved her
perceptions being denied. I asked if this was so. Joanne agreed and went
on to say that she wondered if Chris felt his perception of razors was
being denied by the response of reassurance, which did not directly
address his fears of harming people.

At this point, discussion among the students became animated as they
talked about a different view of Chris' situation. However, further
discussion was interrupted and effectively ended by the entry of a patient
who wanted to know what our meeting was about. When the inter-
ruption had been dealt with, the meeting was at an end.

Although four meetings remained for the students in which to pursue
this particular discussion further, at the next meeting Joanne was absent
on leave, and this delayed any enquiry about her interactions with Chris.

The changing attendance and subjects discussed by the students
hampered the development of cohesion in the discussion group and the
detailed discussion of issues such as those described. The irregular
attendance may have been one factor that contributed to the minimal
differences in attitudes when measures of group A and group B were
compared. Psychiatric patients were perceived similarly by both groups
as lacking control, and being unco-operative, violent and dangerous. A
slight difference showed group A to be less fearful of patients after the
placement than group B. The outcomes seem similar to those of other
studies and could well reflect ingrained attitudes towards psychiatric
patients.

Some findings

At the outset of the research, it was naively hoped that the effect of the
discussions for group A would be demonstrated by a difference between
the postplacement measures of attitude of the two groups. This was not

the case; both groups' attitudes remained broadly similar. This might be evidence of the danger in allowing inexperienced researchers to expend time and resources, both of others and themselves! However, other considerations can be examined in the light of the context of the discussions of group A.

For example, group A's discussions highlighted a theory–practice gap, namely the timing of the examination on general physical nursing during the mental health placement. Educationalists need to attend to the detail of planning courses to ensure a match between the demands of theory and the practical experience in which students are engaged. As a means of learning about and internalizing students' views of their education, group A's discussions were highly effective in illuminating, for the educationalist, the themes, especially the failings, in a course curriculum.

Several of the themes are evident in the above extract of the discussions, particularly the category 'perception of own abilities'. At other meetings, students said they 'couldn't help', 'don't know what to say', 'patients need counsellors', and as here, 'we are not experts'. At one level, this appears to be a lack of confidence in relating to individuals who are suffering from mental illness. It also suggests the sense of vulnerability of these students in relation to other students on diploma and degree courses. The pursuit of higher academic qualifications by nursing as a professional body may result in individual nurses feeling unskilled and unqualified in their practice, believing the experts are elsewhere, and having diplomas and degrees. At another level, references to the need for counsellors and to students not being experts, may be indicative of a continuing desire to split the nurse–patient relationship into discrete tasks. In this instance, counsellors and experts would take on the task of dealing with Chris' fears about razor blades, allowing students to avoid the distress of relating to him. The distress of engaging with the individual would be dealt with by the activity of referring Chris elsewhere and so appearing to do something.

There are other possible contributions to the students' experience. Melia (1987) notes the wealth of literature encouraging communication with patients, often couched as exhortations that nurses should communicate. Exhortation ignores the possibility that lack of communication could indicate a need to defend against the anxiety and uncertainty inherent in nurses' work. Fabricius (1991) draws attention to the struggles that student nurses may have, in their own right, in developing as individuals. In the discussion group, it was striking how often young patients and their problems were a focus. Contact with the problems of others, particularly young people, can be especially distressing for students who may identify directly with the struggles. This may increase a need for students to avoid communicating with such individual patients and the thoughts and feelings they provoke.

The teacher's role in discussion

When teachers use discussion groups in working with students, they are likely to experience discomfort as they hear accounts that describe a very different reality from that hoped for by the teacher. Teachers are reported to respond to this discomfort by adopting a teaching role (McCaugherty, 1991b; Dartington, 1993). The teaching role consists of telling students about what practice should be as indicated by theory. By teaching, it is also possible to defend against the feeling of hopelessness and powerlessness that may be invoked by listening to the students' accounts of distress. The outcome in both instances is the avoidance of distress by the teacher. There is a parallel with the actions of the students in avoiding distress but the essential effect remains the same, as the focus is shifted from the needs of the patients and the needs of students.

The difficulty of listening to painful experiences should not be underestimated. However, it does appear that one way to help students is to provide a framework in which they can share and investigate their experience of nurse–patient relationships and begin to understand the distress encountered and formulate effective responses. The framework proposed here would be to build upon the work from adult learning, experiential learning and reflection by making the focus the relationship between the nurse and the patient. Developing such a framework does not dismiss the pursuit of academic qualification and the necessary motor skills required by professional practitioners. Rather, it would enable the exercise of theory and its application more effectively in the swampy lowlands (Schon, 1987) of interpersonal relationships. There is a risk here of merely exhorting teachers to undertake this work as we now exhort students (Melia, 1987). The difficult problems will not be resolved, only relocated.

A contribution to a solution may arise from thinking of the limitations of the work described here. The discussion group was evidently novel to the students. The level of attendance referred to and statements of the nature of the discussion as a 'chance for a chat', suggest that the discussion group was seen as being peripheral to their overall experience. However, this related to the one-off nature of the discussion group provided. It may be useful to consider whether such an experience could be made more central to the education of nurses and other helping professions. This would recognize the need to support individual practitioners whose work requires the active engagement in interpersonal relationships. Given the reservations described above, such a solution cannot rely only on the individual or a small group of individuals, but demands the attention of nurses and educationalists as a whole to ensure the integration of a focus on relationships and the associated distress this may arouse.

Conclusion

While certificate-level preparatory courses of the type these students attended have now ceased, there remains a need to try to address the issues discussed in this work. Students of nursing, nurses and other professional workers can be expected to encounter such relationship difficulties as described here and struggle with the feelings that are raised.

Supporting the examination of working relationships may be of benefit to students, nurses, teachers and, ultimately, patients by providing a space to discuss the problems and uncertainties of practice and illuminate ways of response. A disparity between theory and practice may be inevitable, as the necessarily abstract conceptualization of theory can never match all the possible practice situations. However, in this instance, a change in the timing of either the placement or the assessment would have allowed greater attention by the student to the aims of the mental health placement. This is not to say that student responses all would have been different, but attention to the structure of education is a prerequisite in supporting a focus on the relationships of students with patients. This could then foster a sense of working together, which would help to counter the isolation experienced by students, patients and teachers in their everyday work.

References

Atkins, S. and Murphy, K. (1993). Reflection: a review of the literature. *J. Adv. Nurs.*, **18**, 1188–1192.
Balint, M. (1957). *The Doctor, His Patient and the Illness*. Tavistock Publications.

Bendall, E. (1975). *So You Passed, Nurse?* Royal College of Nursing.

Boydell, T. (1976). *Experiential Learning*, p. 24, Manchester Monographs.

Burnard, P. (1989). Experiential learning and andrology-negotiated learning in nurse education: a critical appraisal. *Nurse Educ. Today*, 9, 300–306.

Burnard, P. (1991). A method of analysing interview transcripts in quantitative research. *Nurse Educ. Today*, 11, 461–466.

Collister, B. (1983). The value of psychiatric experience in general nurse training [occasional paper]. *Nurs. Times*, 79(29), 66–69.

Coutts-Jarman, J. (1993). Using reflection and experience in nurse education. *Br. J. Nurs.*, 2(1), 77–80.

Crotty, M. (1993). The changing role of the nurse teacher. *Nurse Educ. Today*, 13, 415–420.

Crotty, M. and Butterworth, T. (1992). The emerging role of the nurse teacher in Project 2000 programmes in England: a literature review. *J. Adv. Nurs.*, 17, 1377–1387.

Dartington, A. (1993). Where angels fear to tread. *Winnicott Stud. J. Squiggle Found.*, 7 (Spring), 21–41.

Fabricius, J. (1991). Learning to work with feelings – psychodynamic understanding and small group work with junior student nurses. *Nurse Educ. Today*, 11, 134–142.

General Nursing Council for England and Wales. (1977). *Syllabus for the Certificate of General Nursing*. London.

Gerrish, K. (1992). The nurse teacher's role in the practice setting. *Nurse Educ. Today*, 12, 227–232.

Greenwood, J. (1993). Reflective practice: a critique of the work of Argyris and Schon. *J. Adv. Nurs.*, 18, 1183–1187.

Hawkett, S. (1990). A gap which must be bridged. *Prof. Nurse*, 6, 166–170.

Hinshelwood, R. (1987). *A Dictionary of Kleinian Thought*. Free Association Books.

Jarvis, P. (1992). Theory and practice and the preparation of teachers of nursing. *Nurse Educ. Today*, 12, 258–265.

Jones, J.A. (1985). A study of nurse tutors' conceptualisation of their ward teaching role. *J. Adv. Nurs.*, 10, 349–360.

Kirschenbaum, H. and Henderson, V.L. (1990). *The Carl Rogers Reader*. Constable.

Knowles, M.S. (1980). *The Adult Learner: a Neglected Species*, fourth edition. Gulf.

McCaugherty, D. (1991a). The theory–practice gap in nurse education: its causes and possible solutions. Findings from an action research study. *J. Adv. Nurs.*, 16, 1055–1061.

McCaugherty, D. (1991b). The use of a teaching model to promote reflection and the experiential integration of theory and practice in first-year student nurses: an action research study. *J. Adv. Nurs.*, 16, 534–543.

Melia, K. (1987). *Learning and Working*. Tavistock Publications.

Menzies, I.E.P. (1970). *Social Systems as a Defence Against Anxiety*. Tavistock Publications.

Nolan, M. and Grant, G. (1992). Mid-range theory building and the nursing theory–practice gap: a respite case care study. *J. Adv. Nurs.*, 17, 217–223.

Powell, J.H. (1989). The reflective practitioner in nursing. *J. Adv. Nurs.*, **14**, 824-832.

Procter, N. and Hafner, J. (1991). Student nurses' attitude to psychiatry: the influence of training and personality. *J. Adv. Nurs.*, **16**, 845–849.

Quinn, F.M. (1988). *The Principles and Practice of Nurse Education*, second edition. Croom Helm.

Reed, J. and Procter, N. (1993). *Nurse Education: a Reflective Approach*. Arnold.

Reid, B. (1993). 'But we're doing it already!' Exploring a response to the concept of reflective practice in order to improve its facilitation. *Nurse Educ. Today*, **13**, 305–309.

Schön, D.A. (1983). *The Reflective Practitioner*. Basic Books.

Schön, D.A. (1987). *Educating the Reflective Practitioner*. Jossey Bass.

Schön, D.A. (1991). *The Reflective Teacher*. College Press.

Scott, J. (1990). *The Effect of Clinical Psychiatric Ward Experiences on Student Nurses' Personal Constructs in Relation to Mental Illness* [dissertation]. City University of London.

Webster, R. (1990). The role of the nurse teacher. *Sen. Nurse*, **10**(6), 21–22.

Wilkinson, D. (1982). The effects of brief psychiatric training on the attitudes of general nursing students to psychiatric patients. *J. Adv. Nurs.*, **7**, 239–253.

Chapter 13
Biographical work with older people

Diane Wells

Autobiographies are often cherished possessions in later life. Many older people enjoy telling stories from their past and, if such tales vary over time, this may be a way of 'keeping the biography in good repair' (Johnson, 1991). When health-care workers take an interest in these accounts, the care offered is more likely to incorporate the patients' values and meanings.

This chapter will draw on the author's experience of conducting a course called Biographical Approaches to Working with Older People at the Joint Faculty of Healthcare Science, Kingston University and St George's Medical School, London University. The course forms part of the English National Board course, Nursing Elderly People. It is designed for registered nurses who are employed in community or institutional settings, and working with patients who are experiencing either mental health or physical problems. The course has two main components: literature seminars and Balint-style seminars (Balint, 1957; Balint, et al. 1993).

In the first component, course members study a selection of writings which demonstrate different perspectives on biographical work. Many gerontologists, psychologists and sociologists have recommended that professionals should listen to the stories of older people, both for the development of theory and the improvement of practice. This chapter begins by reviewing three themes in the literature on these biographical approaches. The first is concerned with forming an authentic picture of a person and his or her past (Johnson, 1991). The second is about helping the older person to review and come to terms with his or her life (Butler, 1963; Erikson *et al.*, 1986), and the third, to understand an older person's abilities, and patterns of self management. (Erikson *et al.*, 1986; di Gregorio, 1987).

In the second component, Balint-style seminars (Balint, et al. 1993) enable course members to discuss their relationships with their patients. These seminars provide nurses with time to express their feelings and to gain some theoretical understanding of these relationships. This seems to be necessary if nurses are to develop therapeutic alliances with their patients. Frequently, nurses want to discuss patients who are 'difficult to nurse'. As the nurses tell their stories, they may be able to clarify thoughts and feelings which, until that point, have been latent in their work.

Biographical approaches: three themes from the literature

Gaining an authentic picture of an older person

One of the main proponents of this way of working is Malcolm Johnson (1991). He suggests that health-care workers have been influenced by medicine and social science, each of which take a 'decremental view' of later life. According to biomedicine, older people are less strong and less able to function physiologically than in their younger days. This view has been transferred into much of the psychology used in medicine. Similarly, social science has described the position of older people in society as one of reduced power and status, with more social problems. Johnson does not deny the value of the data produced by these professions, but he points out how such information is a lopsided view which provides us with a dismal picture of old age.

Older people, he suggests, may not perceive life from the same viewpoint as professionals, and so, to gain a more authentic picture, workers need to listen to their clients' stories. He explains that the events chosen and the manner of telling the story will reveal much about the person. Such knowledge helps the worker both to give appropriate care and to support the client in decision making. This is individualized care without assumptions.

Offering a therapeutic opportunity to review life

Many writers have emphasized the therapeutic opportunity that is available in biographical work. Butler (1963) wrote about the naturally occurring phenomenon of life review, by which he meant the wish to revisit the past in thought and to come to terms with it. He worked with many older people who had become sad, anxious and dysfunctional in later life, but, when given an opportunity to talk about their lives with an interested professional over a period of weeks or months, they often regained a sense of identity and strength. Butler thought that everyone has a need for this sort of review, and that many care-workers can provide the opportunity and support that may be needed.

This idea of life review is similar to Erikson's theory about the last stage of psychosocial development, in which older people may gain a sense of integrity if they can come to terms with the life lived. When this is not possible, and the older person is full of regrets, anger or remorse, then they may be left with a sense of despair. Coleman (1986) developed this by studying the phenomena of those who find satisfaction through reminiscence, and those who find it too painful; the latter are in a minority, but it is important for practitioners to be aware of this group.

Perceiving the recurring patterns in people's lives

The third group of writers encourage us to look for emergent patterns that develop through the lifespan. Erikson's (1950) theory of personality development depicts eight stages from babyhood to old age. Each stage of life is experienced through the self already developed, and so each task is viewed as if through spectacles which retain lenses tinted by past experiences. It is not so much a list of achievements to be ticked off before going on to the next, but rather of being interested in the nature of people's capacities to hope, love, work or be independent, and in how these facets interact.

A more recent researcher, the sociologist di Gregorio (1987), listened to the accounts of a group of older people in Leeds, and then, by using their concept of 'managing', elucidated their patterns of managing. The patterns that emerged were remarkably consistent through the lifespan. For example, a woman who had looked to her family for support in early life would continue this pattern into old age. Similarly, one who insisted on functioning independently in her youth usually retained this pattern in later life.

Balint-style seminars: some examples

These writings provide the nurses undertaking the course with some ideas to support their biographical work with patients. The Balint-style seminars are an opportunity to develop this aspect of the work. For example, while recapturing and retelling their own experiences, nurses remember and realize their own competence, as well as their own omissions. No-one can tell a person how to feel or how to act in relationships, and yet, insight gained through discussion can help nurses to perceive what has happened in the past and to consider the future. Four examples of work with patients are described below.

Mrs R and Angela

Mrs R was in hospital for investigations because she had been unable to eat, and for several weeks had felt nauseous and weak. Angela, her nurse, spent long periods talking with her about what she might eat, and trying to coax her with tasty morsels, soft food and refreshing drinks. Angela also talked with Mrs R about her life, and came to know how important her son was to her, especially since the death of her husband two or three years earlier. Many medical investigations were carried out; nothing conclusive was found. Angela described to the seminar group how the notes were getting fatter whilst the patient was getting thinner! Then Angela thought, 'I have not seen this son; does he visit when I am not here?' On asking her patient, she learnt that the son had fairly recently become disabled, used a wheelchair, and had been unable to visit his mother. 'I am sure we can arrange something,' said Angela, and set about making arrangements for appropriate transport to bring the son to his mother. A few days later, Angela was trying to coax Mrs R with yoghurt again. After two spoonfuls, Mrs R thought it was enough; then Angela was aware of a wheelchair drawing up at her side, and a voice said, 'Give me that, nurse. I'll help Mum.' Once Mrs R and her son were together and talking, she found swallowing was easy. Arrangements were made for the son to visit regularly, and Mrs R's digestive problems subsided. She regained her weight, but she still seemed to require a great deal of attention from the nurses. One day, Mrs R called 'Angela can you come?' Angela went, and Mrs R pointed to the ground saying 'Look there's a pea on the floor. Would you pick it up?' Angela had explained to her on several occasions how busy the ward was, and this was almost too much.

Nevertheless, she picked it up, saying again how much work there was to be done. She pondered on the reasons for Mrs R's behaviour. Why was she continuing to ask for help when nothing was required, and she was better anyway. Angela decided she could not take this behaviour any more, and so she avoided Mrs R whenever she could. Mrs R was almost ready for discharge, and, as this time got nearer, Angela felt increasingly unhappy about the distance she felt she had created between them. Before leaving, Mrs R called Angela to her side, and said, 'Thank you nurse. You know you have been more than a nurse to me.' Angela felt glad that her work had been appreciated after all, and very moved that her patient had instigated this warm farewell.

Angela had discussed these events in the course seminars on several occasions. After the discharge, Angela reviewed her nursing of Mrs R, and began to see patterns in Mrs R's relationships. It seemed that she had been quite dependent on her husband; when he died, this dependency seemed to have been transferred to the son. It was when the son became disabled that Mrs R was unable to eat. The eating difficulties and her frequent requests for help could be understood as attempts to recreate a situation where she could be dependent and receive help as she had in the past, first from her husband, and then from her son. Angela thought this idea was the key to her relationship with Mrs R. If only she had understood this earlier, she thought, she need not have created the distance between them; but then, Mrs R may not have instigated the warm goodbye, which was an independent act, quite different from her earlier behaviour to Angela, and probably therapeutic for Mrs R.

Rachel and Helen

While working as a night nurse, Rachel had one very ill patient, Helen, who probably did not have very long to live. Rachel had nursed many people in their last weeks of life, but this situation was very different. When Rachel was a child, Helen had lived nearby and, as a family friend, had helped Rachel to dress her dolls and take them out for walks. Helen had been an important carer for the nurse when she was a child; now everything had been turned around. They had not seen one another for years, so meeting in these circumstances gave Rachel mixed feelings of pain and joy. Helen needed a lot of care, which Rachel was glad to give, but Rachel could not bring herself to talk about their shared memories. She was not clear about what was stopping her; after all, she wanted to tell Helen about the valuable memories she had of the time they had spent together. Having thought, read and talked about it in the seminars, eventually one night Rachel said to Helen, 'I remember how you used to help me dress my dolls . . . ' Then the conversation flowed, as each remembered and stimulated memories in the other.

Nursing Helen had been difficult and sad, and at the same time very rewarding, both professionally and personally. It had been a most unusual experience, but it had given Rachel the confidence to respond to another patient's need to reminisce.

Rachel and Mrs O

Rachel was working on Christmas morning and was very concerned about Mrs O, who was very weak, in pain, and probably had only a few days to live. She had been given her usual analgesia, but it had not had its usual effect that day. 'Mother!' called out Mrs O. Rachel knew her mother had died years ago, but she went to the bedside and asked, 'Was she a good woman, your mother?' There was a look of relief on Mrs O's face, as Rachel sat down, took her hand, and decided that this was the important work for the next-however-long-it-took. Mrs O talked about how her mother used to play the piano, and what she remembered singing at Christmas. Rachel asked about her father, and the other members of the family. Mrs O talked about them, and then about the games they played and the few toys they had. She described it as a 'good childhood' and settled down to rest; this was clearly the best form of analgesia. Mrs O died peacefully the next day.

Jane and Mrs T

Jane was nursing Mrs T, who was recovering from a stroke. Mrs T was very enthusiastic about her rehabilitation programme, but insisted that nurses should do things in certain ways to help her. She wanted her belongings and hospital furniture to be placed exactly as she required, so that she could be as independent as possible. The nurses sometimes found this a bit tiresome, particularly because Mrs T would watch to see if they placed things where she needed them to be. If they were not in the right place, Mrs T would point it out and ask for them to be changed. She was not unpleasant, but the nurses were beginning to label her as 'demanding'.

While helping her with everyday activities, Jane talked with Mrs T about her life. She came to understand how Mrs T had always been very independent. Her parents had always encouraged her to make up her own mind, and not to depend on others. Even now, despite her disabilities, she felt determined to make these 'tree-trunk stiff legs', as she called them, work again. The future she envisaged was back in her own flat, with her dog for company. Jane had always been sympathetic to Mrs T's viewpoint, but, armed with this evidence, Jane hoped to convince her colleagues that Mrs T was not merely 'demanding'. Jane presented her case, and her colleagues said yes, they understood. The nurses became a little more responsive to Mrs T's precise instructions, but when their patience ran out, as at times it did, there were complaints, not only about Mrs T's demands but also about the way Jane seemed to support her behaviour. Jane was convinced that her response to Mrs T was appropriate, especially as her patient slowly improved. Eventually, Mrs T was well enough to manage again in her small flat, although she had to surrender the care of her dog to someone else. Jane shared Mrs T's joy about going home and her sadness at losing her dog. Jane herself felt sad about the gulf that was sometimes present between herself and her colleagues in relation to Mrs T's care.

Reviewing the examples with course members

In each of these situations, a knowledge of the patient's biography was an important element. Each nurse, through her interest in biographies and a willingness to be involved with her patients, achieved some success in nursing.

Angela helped Mrs R to see her son instead of having more medical investigations for her symptoms. The experience with Angela probably also helped Mrs R to take a step towards independence. This happened because Angela took an interest in Mrs R's family, her past and present relationships, and her patterns of managing. This supports di Gregorio's (1987) idea that people repeat their patterns of management throughout their lives.

I showed Angela what I had written in this chapter about her nursing of Mrs R. She was reminded of how angry she had felt with this patient, and she added:

> Angry with myself, I couldn't understand her not eating; there was no medical diagnosis. Then later, when I had done all this work, and still she said things like: 'Could you pick up that pea?'

I asked Angela what had encouraged her to do all this work, and she replied:

Before the course, it [nursing] tended to be physical, but doing the course helped me to understand the importance of relationships and life stories: to go into detail about people's earlier lives, their relationships, their ways of coping with losses, who helped, and then seeing what relevance that had for nursing.

When I asked what difference that has made to her nursing now, she said:

If you have time at the beginning to make a relationship, it helps. We need more staff. But sometimes it helps me understand. We have a woman who has lost her speech after a stroke. She likes watching television, but we could not understand what she was indicating. When I asked the family, they explained that she has been a keen golf player, and is happiest when she can watch golf. Times like this – it comes – we understand, but I wish I could spend more time. Now, I do think if a person behaves in an awkward manner, there may be a reason.

We have a male patient now who can be very particular; but I ask him about his past life and we discuss it, and I think he feels younger, and is reminded of times when he was more independent. Then it's more possible to work with him. The course gave me a boost to understanding relationships, why people find things difficult. There was time to acknowledge how awkward things are, and time to understand.

Because Rachel already knew quite a lot about Helen's early life, and was aware that Helen did not have long to live, Rachel wanted to support and share in her life review (Butler, 1963; Erikson et al., 1986). Although this was difficult, Rachel did it, and demonstrated very clearly the emotional cost and satisfaction for herself. Once 'over the hump', Rachel felt freer to offer another patient, Mrs O, an opportunity to reminisce on Christmas morning, and this turned out to be the best form of pain relief.

Rachel's memories of the course also included the idea of a place where one could discuss dreadful experiences, consider solutions and, if that did not work, return for another discussion. During the course, she had taken on a new role, and the opportunities for discussion had helped her develop her own management style. She explained how, if staff see her taking an interest in people's lives, they do too:

It's a much more rounded and softer approach to nursing, but some who wanted more routine to the way they work have left. This morning we were talking about a patient and his relatives; the staff enjoy it, but we can't spend a lot of time.

I asked if there were any problems. 'Yes,' said Rachel, 'we need to be friendly, not familiar. There is a dividing line, and if we step over it we're in trouble. The nurses know this.' The implication was 'we have to be vigilant'.

Jane's example showed how her understanding and empathy developed from hearing how Mrs T had lived her life. Jane wanted to understand Mrs T's viewpoint, and saw this understanding as an essential aspect of the rehabilitation programme. The other nurses, who were less motivated to understand Mrs T's point of view, were also less sympathetic.

When Jane read my account of her work with Mrs T, she said:

> The rehabilitation programme with this lady was so long, the progress was very slow. It was a major piece of work supporting her, and getting to know how she had lived her life was difficult because it was not considered by colleagues to be a worthy task.

'What about Mrs T?' I asked, 'What did she think?'

> Oh, she liked our chats, and without understanding her like that and seeing her point of view, I could not have helped her so much. It raised her self-esteem, and then she could do more. Looking back, it was a valuable piece of work and now that I work for social services, I use these skills of getting to know how someone has lived their life a lot. But in a ward, when working as a nurse, there's a culture that says 'hurry up', and you have to fit in. You're trying to keep everyone happy, and that makes it very difficult to do the sort of work I did with Mrs T. My colleagues did not understand, I think, because they did not have the knowledge to help them understand.

I agreed that it is difficult to make changes within an organization unless others want that change also. I then asked her what had happened to Mrs T. Jane said:

> I saw her two or three months after she was discharged; she was still in her flat, and it was hard for her, but she was glad to be there and enjoying the spring flowers.

Conclusion

These examples show how nurses can increase their therapeutic impact by knowing something of their patients' life stories. Biographical knowledge, however, is not enough; it is the relationship between the nurse and the patient that is the crucial factor. It is here that the nurse experiences tensions, responds to needs or gives support. When attention is paid to the emotional aspects of getting to know patients, nurses are best able to use a biographical approach in their care of patients.

References

Balint, E., Courtnay, M., Elder, A., Hull, S. and Julian, P. (1993). *The Doctor, the Patient and the Group*. Routledge.

Balint, M. (1968). *The Doctor, His Patient, and the Illness*, revised second edition. Pitman Paperbacks.

Butler, R.N. (1963). The life review: an interpretation of reminiscence in the aged. *Psychiatry*, 26, 65–76.

Coleman, P. (1986). *Ageing and Reminiscence Processes*. John Wiley.

di Gregorio, S. (1987). *Social Gerontology: New Directions*. Croom Helm.

Erikson, E.H. (1950). *Childhood and Society*. Norton.

Erikson, E.H., Erikson, J.M. and Kivnick, H.Q. (1986). *Vital Involvement in Old Age*. Norton.

Johnson, M. (1991). The meaning of old age. In *Nursing Elderly People* (S. Redfern, ed.) Second edn. pp. 3–17, Churchill Livingstone.

Further reading

Birren, J.E., Kenyon, G.M., Ruth, J.E. *et al*. eds. (1996). Aging and Biography: Explorations in Adult Development. Springer Publishing Company Inc.

Chapter 14
Clinical supervision

Mic Rafferty

This chapter is concerned with clinical supervision, both as a concept, and as professional and personal experience. The illustrations and observations are drawn from participants on programmes run by the Department of Nursing, Midwifery and Health Care at University College Swansea. The programmes prepare nurses and health visitors, first to identify their own needs for supervision, and then to begin the process of developing the skills they will need to supervise others (Rafferty and Coleman, 1996). The programmes aim to model good supervisory practice through their structures and processes, so that participants can experience for themselves what it is like to receive supervision. The programmes provide many opportunities for participants to reflect on the way they work, to discover and make explicit the knowledge and skills which they take for granted, and the practices which have become unthinking routine.

My role as educational manager of these programmes enables me to work with nurses concerning what is supervision, and how it might be conducted. Such work has made it clear to me that supervision is something many nurses long for. In the programmes we offer, they see, at last, a chance to give serious attention to their practice of care. They quickly grasp the benefits of being able to pay attention to their professional and personal joys and sorrows, and the complexities and responsibilities of their craft.

To give an example, Gemma, an experienced staff nurse in the care of the aged, described how she had recently transferred to a ward specializing in the medical treatment of respiratory disorders. On recognizing her lack of expertise in this specialty, she entered into a supervisory relationship with the respiratory nurse specialist, Joan. With Joan, Gemma reviewed the therapeutic reasons that determine practice for a patient in her care, in particular, the administration of bronchodilators through the use of a nebulizer. Gemma was appalled to discover that, when nursing the aged, she was failing to follow recommendations related to correct humidification. This meant less than optimal delivery of medication, inaccurate peak flow measurements, and, possibly, slower recovery.

While upholding Gemma's accountability for her actions, we should recognize that this opportunity for supervision by a specialist practitioner is uncommon. Accountability can be reasonably expected only when nurses have regular opportunities in practice to anticipate, explain and justify their judgements and actions.

Michael, a mental health nurse of some experience, was trying to get to grips again with general nursing. To achieve this, he worked two shifts a month as a staff nurse in an elderly care setting. On a morning shift, after assisting David to eat, wash and dress for the day, Michael noticed he was becoming increasingly sad and withdrawn. Michael, following conversations with David and drawing upon what he knew and thought to be important, judged this response as a reaction to a long period of hospitalization and, in particular, to missing his dog, Bess. Michael failed to recognize that David's withdrawal was due to his being in physical pain. It took the knowledge of another nurse, at a later stage, for Michael to realize this.

It was obvious to Jean, the ward sister, that all was not right in the working relationship between the mother of Sam, who had been admitted for a tonsillectomy, and Brenda, the primary nurse. The disdain was mutual, and the tension in the relationship was palpable. Jean worried about how this would impact upon the postoperative care of Sam, but did not feel able to draw Brenda's attention to the disharmony, or try to provide Brenda with the means to deal with it. The day after the operation, Brenda forgot to follow – until reminded – the ward protocol, which allowed children to take fluids after recovery from an anaesthetic.

Implicit in these stories is the uncomfortable fact that nurses sometimes make errors in their clinical judgements. Even more disturbing, the Allitt Inquiry (1991) forced public and professional attention to the truth that nurses can, and sometimes do, cause deliberate harm to those in their care. Complaints by patients and their relatives indicate that nurses can, on occasions, be thoughtless, provocative and mean-minded in the care they give.

If nurses are to respond sensitively to the needs of their patients, it is essential that they should have opportunities to understand their own responses to them. The giving of self – the crucial dimension of care – has to be supported, nurtured and guarded. This giving of self requires the capacity to be both empathic and sympathetic, the ability to be vulnerable to the experience of others. This is where clinical supervision becomes important.

What is clinical supervision?

Winnicott's (1965) concept of 'holding', provides a useful way of understanding the supervisory function. Holding is about providing a developmentally appropriate environment, one which protects against harm, provides a context that promotes sensitivity to another's condition, and allows for individuation and the need for growth and development.

Holding in supervision is primarily about preventing physiological harm to the patient by attending to the nurse's needs for professional support, practice learning and opportunities to ensure accountability. The emphasis on the physical is not to ignore the psychosocial aspects of care, but to stress the crucial relationship between emotional and social experience, and physical wellbeing.

The core of effective supervision is to help the clinical practitioner to make sense of the experience of caring. It is about providing regular opportunities for nurses to explore what they can realistically do or not do, or prevent or not prevent, so that expectations that protect the nurse and the patient may be clarified and agreed.

Supervision and support

Providing care can be at profound personal cost to nurses. A nurse who has established a warm and mutually valued working relationship with a patient undergoing renal dialysis, twice weekly, year in year out, is bound to be affected by the patient's slow decline and death. Special care baby nurses, who bond with premature babies and struggle with all their technical, intuitive and caring might, to keep them alive, can be shattered by the baby's survival in a desperately crippled state. The accident and emergency sister, who has witnessed five deaths in one shift, has to be deeply troubled. Such personal experiences confront nurses with dilemmas about the point of their work, and provoke emotions that are usual in experiences of loss and grief. Such situations, which tax our abilities to cope as care-workers, can cause us to suffer from stress and burnout. This can produce sickness, anxiety or depression, and ways of coping which are potentially harmful, such as cigarette smoking or the excessive consumption of alcohol.

Opportunities to feel grief, disgust and hopelessness, as well as pleasure, attractiveness and possibilities, help nurses to recognize and respond appropriately to the here-and-now of their work environment. They can begin to see the story of their everyday work, and its implications for them and their patients. Valuing emotional experience makes it possible to recognize and work with moral dilemmas.

Nurses have for too long been denied appropriate opportunities to recognize and work with their emotional experience. When, during the supervisory course, nurses are given opportunities to reflect upon a practice experience, they often choose to explore a painful incident which raises doubts about what they did. The fact that such events are frequently long past suggests that nurses can be haunted by the ghosts of what they have done or seen in their professional life.

Particular trouble arises when nurses feel they are the cause of harm; when they make mistakes, for instance, or fail to notice, anticipate, or interpret correctly a fateful change or event, as the examples above illustrate. The suicide of a patient, for a community mental health nurse, is frequently a devastating experience. Afterwards, it is not unusual to find the nurse preoccupied with the event and intent on remembering conversations with the client, searching for what might have been missed. General nurses involved in drastic therapeutic practice can feel a sense of being harmful. For instance: caring for elderly patients who undergo repeated amputations aimed at halting tissue necrosis; or caring for patients with leukaemia, where the chemotherapy battle is fought to the bitter, and what often seems inevitable, end. Health visitors and school nurses have to deal with their potential to be harmful when their professional accountability demands that they act on a child's report of sexual abuse, leading to potential disintegration of the family.

Nurses, as a result of experiences associated with harm, usually react with appropriate feelings, which include anger, shame and embarrassment. They also can be quite irrationally guilt-ridden, with a distorted sense of their own responsibility and a loss of capacity for work.

That such harm can be held, worked with, and learnt from, is a difficult idea for some nurses to accept, because the ideal of altruistic giving and correctness is central to our socialization. The problem is compounded by institutional responses to mistakes in practice, which are frequently experienced as punitive and unfair.

Supervision, because it is about everyday practice, allows nurses to attend to what they do that is right, as well as wrong. This provides much needed opportunities for good practice to be recognized and affirmed, and allows omissions and mistakes to be kept in proportion. Supervisory relationships in which the nurse feels connected, understood and purposeful, give opportunities to identify and own grey areas of practice. They enable nurses to do the right thing, and, if necessary, make reparation.

Personal and professional lives

Louise, a student nurse, is undertaking a placement in a general practice ward of a community hospital. During an evening shift, she assists with the admission of a middle-aged man, who is unconscious and critically ill after a subarachnoid haemorrhage. Louise has to deal with this man's distraught wife and children. She tries to emulate the behaviour of other nurses, who are efficient, professional and seemingly resigned to the fact that this patient will die. Louise's boyfriend had died a year earlier following a subarachnoid haemorrhage. She keeps in check her own feeling of sadness and numbness about what is happening. After the rest of the shift has passed in an 'inefficient fog', she goes home and spends the night crying, alone, in sadness and despair. Louise would be the first to claim the other nurses were genuinely interested in providing support and learning opportunities, but no-one else talked about the personal implications of care for them, so how could she? Like them, she took her troubles home with her.

Nurses can experience unbearable tensions when there is too great a resonance between their private life and their professional work. Issues can range from not being able to have children, for a nurse working with patients having a termination of pregnancy, to caring for a patient when a loved one is dying, or, as in Louise's case, has died of the same illness. Frequently, due to lack of opportunities to address the distress, the only solution is to leave the job, or to change clinical areas. When adequate supervisory relationships are in place, however, it is possible to sustain a nurse through such a time of crisis. This means listening to and valuing the emotional world of the nurse, helping him or her to use others who are seen as supportive, and giving encouragement to continue with any work or leisure activities the nurse feels able to do. While counselling and occupational health have a place for nurses experiencing long-term emotional distress, in the first instance the most effective help comes from a supervisor who can be relied upon to listen.

Learning from practice

Weddell (1968a: p. 20) asserts that nurses must be able to examine and criticize their own and other nurses' practice, without blame or scapegoating, in order to learn. Unfortunately, my experience supports Butterworth's (1992: p. 13) observation that nursing case conferences are a rare event. Out of the 100 nurses who have attended the supervision modules at Swansea, only a handful had had opportunities to make presentations of work for peer review. Nurses, whose practice spanned neonatal to elderly care, and included representatives from every role within hospital and community health services, were rarely given more than a few minutes to talk about the care that they gave. In hospital settings, shift handovers – so vital for continuity and problem identification – are usually experienced as a race against time, and as a battle to keep distractions in check. This state of affairs represents the current reality of supervision in nursing, and points to the challenges that have to be overcome.

Without supervisory opportunities to present their work, newly qualified nurses find it hard to develop abilities to demonstrate an argument, assert a perspective, summarize, or engage in collaborative problem solving. The lack of such presentational skills has serious implications for patient care. Whale (1993) found that the nursing contribution to a multidisciplinary ward round was more likely to be determined by the chairmanship of the doctor, rather than the nurse's knowledge of patients' needs and problems. This was due to lack of confidence, assertiveness and abilities to present a nursing perspective.

The numerous difficult and painful interactions with medical staff recalled by nurses provide further justification for supporting them so that they can deal with the personal consequences of being bullied, ridiculed and patronized, as well as spending time developing assertiveness and conflict-management techniques.

Another reason for attending to practice learning is to make use of a precious nursing resource, practice knowledge. The clinical accounts of nurses indicate that they take for granted and regard as unremarkable what they know. Often, nurses assume their knowledge is obvious and self-evident, because they rarely talk about it in any detail. Part of the problem lies in the fact that nursing is a practice discipline which, out of necessity, has to value doing. No matter how complex the doing is, it inevitably becomes routine. Routine leads to familiarity and familiarity to the absence of obvious thoughtfulness.

The experiences of nurses suggests that we still have a culture of learning from watching, rather than also talking about what was done and why it was done, based upon the evidence of effectiveness. Without opportunities to present accounts of care, the enormous complexity of nursing will continue to be unappreciated.

Rachel, who attended one of the supervision modules, told how she had taken seriously the challenge to listen to the language she used in practice, and to attend to her own experience of providing care. She recalled with embarrassment how she heard herself telling another nurse to get a bed ready for the admission of a 'smelly big toe'. Reflecting upon the words she used, she recognized how difficult she found it to care for patients with vascular insufficiency to the limbs. The 'smelly toe', over the years, became the 'smelly foot', then ankle, then calf, then leg. The patient's constant pain would be interspaced by periods of more acute pain following operation after operation, in a vain attempt to stop tissue necrosis. The patient's death seemed inevitable. Rachel identified that many similar experiences with such patients had become too much for her, and so she went out of her way to avoid any real engagement with them. Supervisory help to reflect on her experience, however, had made a difference this time. Rather than keeping away from this man, she now responded to his curiosity about how circulation was affected by diet. Her advice was obviously heeded, for the man returned to the ward after attending outpatients, to show off the much improved circulation to his big toe.

Ensuring accountability: the appropriate use of authority

Weddell (1968b: p. 241) calls for an administrative structure in nursing which gives security by encouraging initiative and creativity within known limits. Implicit in this structure is the idea of appropriate supervisory authority (Hawkins and Shohet, 1989: p. 39). Course members, in discussing issues of authority in supervision, raise a variety of issues, ranging from unease about setting standards for peers, to problems in persuading colleagues to acknowledge and change ineffective practice. Accountability, in the context of supervision, is about providing nurses with opportunities to justify their professional judgements. This function is contentious, because too often nurses feel scrutinized and controlled by someone whose authority is based on position rather than knowledge. Nurses are concerned that supervision can become just one more way to gain compliance, rather than an opportunity to have accountability affirmed.

As part of the course, we demonstrate how mutually agreed contracts between the supervisor and the supervisee can establish a shared quality control element. Supervision can then become a helpful and safe opportunity to show how professional judgements and actions were determined. The clinically knowledgeable supervisor is in the best position to offer advice and guidance about therapeutic knowledge, and organizational and professional norms; an emphasis on practice reasoning gives mutual opportunities for good practice to be affirmed, shortcomings to be identified, and corrective or protective measures to be agreed. Given the right conditions, nurses will willingly engage in opportunities to be called to account for their practice and accept that *accountable* practice is *examined* practice.

Many of the issues brought to the course are about difficult and problematic professional relationships. A recurrent theme is nurses feeling exasperated, ill-used and let down by colleagues for whom they have supervisory responsibilities. These colleagues are often experienced as hopeless and beyond redemption, to be got rid of, if possible, or punished. Such responses support Hawthorne's (1975) finding that the wish to abdicate, or to manipulate their position power, are common problems for supervisors. Supervisory training and support provide opportunities for this destructive human potential to be kept in check. Supervisors, as well as nurses, need help not to react unthinkingly in response to provocation, but to stay engaged, and continue with finding ways to engage helpfully with those they experience as difficult.

Sian, for example, the elected team leader of a group of school nurses, was charged with establishing a nurse-led immunization programme which was safe and effective. Her colleagues, although well versed with immunization routines, had previously worked under the authority of a medical practitioner. Sian, and other nurses working in an immunization clinic, had been confronted by a series of problems which indicated their failure to prepare adequately for the task. For example, just before commencement, it was discovered that the adrenaline, necessary in case of anaphylactic shock, had passed its use-by date. Although neither she nor the team had ever had to use this drug, she insisted they held up immunization until it had been replaced. The delay was compounded when they discovered that the replacement adrenaline, which had been fetched from the pharmacy, had also passed its expiry date and had to be replaced yet again. At the end of the clinic, Sian was left feeling the other nurses were cross with her about the delay, and dismissive of her as an old fusspot.

In the course setting, Sian recognized how uncomfortable it was for her to use authority. She expressed her worry that others experienced her meticulous attention to detail as evidence of an obsessive compulsive personality, a worry shared by her colleagues. The supervision module provided an opportunity to support Sian about the appropriateness of what she had done, and reassurance that she had exercised authority well in a difficult and personally demanding situation. This enabled Sian to go back to the team and persuade them to reflect collaboratively upon their experience of the immunization clinic. Together, they identified what had to change in team behaviour to ensure good practice in the future.

Conclusion

The experiences of nurses attending a course in supervision have been used to illustrate a compelling and urgent need to help them to sustain and develop their professional practice. Clinical supervision, as we have seen, is about creating conditions and relationships which make it possible to examine the logic behind the doing, to verify its appropriateness, and to manage the giving of self in order to protect both the patient and the nurse. Supervision provides ongoing opportunities to check that the care offered to patients is good enough, and provides nurses with opportunities for support, learning and the exercise of professional accountability. It allows mutual judgements about knowledge, skills and developmental needs, and, in attending to the emotional experiences of nurses, helps to sustain their capacity to give of themselves in extremely distressing circumstances.

Conditions have to be created in practice so that unintentional or possible deliberate harm can be prevented; true consumer protection demands a context in which it is possible to provide, protect and enable safe and effective care. The threats to the ideals of supervision lie not with nurses, who are usually only too glad of the chance to discuss and reflect on their professional practice; they come, rather, from the failure of institutional and professional commitment to those structures and resources that make clinical supervision possible, usual, protected and respected.

References

Butterworth, T. (1992). Clinical supervision as an emerging idea in nursing. In *Clinical Supervision and Mentorship in Nursing* (T. Butterworth and J. Faugier, eds.) pp. 3–17, Chapman and Hall.

Hawkins, P. and Shohet, R. (1989). *Supervision in the Helping Professions.* Open University Press.

Hawthorne, L. (1975). Games supervisors play. *Soc. Work*, (20 May), 179–183.

Kappeli, S. (1987). A matter of definition. *Nurs. Times*, 83(44), 67–69.

The Clothies Report (1994). *The Allitt Inquiry: Independent Inquiry Relating to Deaths and Injuries on the Children's Ward at Grantham and Kesteven General Hospital During the Period February to April 1991.* HMSO.

Rafferty, M.A. and Coleman, M.R. (1996). Educating for clinical supervision. *Nurs. Stand.*, 10(45),38–41.

Weddell, D. (1968a). Outline of nurse training. In *Psychosocial Nursing: Studies from the Cassel Hospital* (E. Barnes, ed.) pp. 16–23, Tavistock Publications.

Weddell, D. (1968b). Human relations in nursing administration. In *Psychosocial Nursing: Studies from the Cassel Hospital* (E. Barnes, ed.) pp. 231–242, Tavistock Publications.

Whale, Z. (1993). The participation of hospital nurses in the multidisciplinary ward round on a cancer-therapy ward. *J. Clin. Nurs.*, 1, pp. 155–164.

Winnicott, D.W. (1965). *The Theory of the Parent–infant Relationship: The Maturational Process and the Facilitating Environment* pp. 37–55, Hogarth.

Chapter 15

Psychosocial issues of racism in the caring professions: a black perspective

Sonia Stephen

This chapter is dedicated to a recent ancestor, Amos Wilson, black psychologist. May his wisdom, knowledge and brilliance forever shine through those who follow him, in the sure acknowledgement of the importance and significance of his life's work. Hetepu (peace and blessings).

If black people are expected to be themselves and not merely a darkened version of Europeans, race has to be in the consulting rooms, in the corridors and on the staircases of every institution of which black people are a part. The issue of equality and race must be constantly on the agenda, painful though it can be to have to live with the realities of our joint histories.

The issue of blackness and the Cassel Hospital is incongruous. I would like to explore why I think this is so. I start from the position of realizing that this exploration could not have begun if its seeds had not been planted by my experiences at this hospital. I left the Cassel Hospital in 1988, having spent almost five years there, culminating in the post of clinical nurse specialist for the single adults unit, which I held for two years. It must be said that this is a personal exploration, based on my memory of the experience, and as such is a very Afrocentric approach and perspective, not one based on logic; it is an approach realized after leaving the hospital.

My time there was central in the development of my understanding of organizations, how they function and people's roles and identities within them. Once I understood organizational dynamics, and my place within them, the impact of my race on the institution became clear. On leaving the hospital, this self-knowledge, plus the ability to articulate both what I could see and feel, and the skills honed during my time there, served me well as a group psychotherapist, staff-team facilitator, and management consultant in both black and white communities. The ability to challenge the perceived order is essential to the understanding of a black identity. I would like to consider: some of the psychological issues raised by the need for such full cultural assimilation as part of the treatment programme; and the notion of privilege, both within the staff team as well as the patients, and the psychodynamics of the white on black interaction. I would also like to explore the development of the black psyche as a therapeutic tool, and to consider how psychosocial care could be used within the black community.

Why are the Cassel Hospital and blackness incongruous?

Everything about the Cassel is riddled with white middle-classness: its beautiful location sandwiched between Richmond Park, Ham Common, and an expansive garden; its grand entrance, with its sweeping Gloria Swanson staircase; the perfect wooden-floored, double French-windowed dining room; just off the bay-windowed alcove, a common room with ballroom proportions; and several bedrooms that comfortably house four beds. It is almost always in need of some maintenance work and looks slightly frayed and shabby, a relic of a better era, but there is constant hope that, with some attention and care, it could once again shine in its full glory. It seems an almost concrete symbol of the individual struggles, and the hope and fears, of those who work within it.

Not only was it middle-classness expressed in concrete terms, but also in its acknowledgement of its norms. During my time there it had a male-dominated culture. I understand there have been at least two female consultants, but, on the whole, we females appear to have known our places, as lead nurse (matron) and principal child psychotherapist (mother/nurturer). The male-dominated therapy team, 'the doctors', and the female dominated nurse team, 'the nurses', worked together and in parallel. Both were equally significant within their own right and focused on different needs and different roles. This is where I began to understand the fact that 'different' did not mean 'inferior', at least in gender and professional terms.

I became aware that the impact of the nurses and nursing often outstripped that of the doctors. We were based in reality of day-to-day functioning 24 hours a day, in the here and now. The doctors/therapists worked with the internalized world of the there and then, leaving a space (the community) for the nurse to work with the patient about the 'here and now' and how it is affected by the 'there and then'.

The patients' community used the democratic principle for internal organizational decision making. A clear hierarchical structure reflected that of the nurses and doctors within each unit and the community as a whole. There was an acknowledgement of difference and order, and a general agreement that everything within the community was accessible for examination, exploration and analysis. Nothing was incidental or accidental, everything told a story, and everything was interrelated and interdependent. To be able to work within this culture, either as a patient or staff member, requires full cultural assimilation and integration.

To do this as a black person requires one to transcend one's blackness in order to see and experience the world as though one were white. This is not only the case for people engaged in the Cassel experience. This is the case for all nonwhites immersed in the European experience.

The dilemma of European blackness

We came to and stayed in this country during and since the Second World War, with the intention of self-improvement, and the attainment of better education, better job prospects and a future for our children. We were going to the place where rightness, justice, fair play and democracy were born, a place where, once you played the game, worked hard, and kept your nose clean, all things beyond your wildest dreams, including heaven, could be yours. (The close proximity to all that whiteness must surely rub off, and help toward acceptance in the eyes of the white God.)

Due to the internalization of racism, to be successful meant to be as far from black as possible, as far from one's true self as possible, and to identify with the majority community. We often had to operate against our own best interests and in the interest of the Europeans. We have been successfully conditioned not to make white people uncomfortable. Each individual is an ambassador of the entire race and personally responsible for how black people are perceived by the white community. We are socialized to soak up racism without acknowledgement and to do almost anything within our power to maintain the peace and equilibrium, and to absorb negativism, as a duty, if we are to be responsible black people. We could not challenge, we were not even allowed to be aware, but were forced to overlook injustice or to make it a personal issue, as if it was our own fault.

Any black person who had made it as far as the Cassel Hospital, be it as a patient or a member of staff, had to be so far removed from their blackness as to deserve the title I had in the black community of 'Miss English'. The majority black community did not understand me, and I did not understand it. With only a mock sense of self, there can be no integrity. So I, like Europeans, was drawn to psychotherapy in a desperate search for sense and purpose.

Psychoanalysis and psychotherapy are very much a European (white, nineteenth-century) necessity because Europeans have lost connection with their true self. They value science and technology above nature and divinity. It has become almost impossible for them to trust themselves (subjectivism). The truth is now only true if it is qualified, analysed, defined and preferably published! Somehow, this is meant to make it objective (objectivism).

Psychotherapy and psychoanalysis reflect Europeans' scientific attempts to rediscover the true self–spirit–soul without loss of face in terms of objectivity. It is the European's attempt to rediscover the spirit on an individual and group basis. This is what was taken away from the African people, unvalued, by association with blackness (denigrated) and used as part justification for their use and abuse for centuries. The black person's relationship with the indwelling spirit and the spirit of those who have gone before us, along with the acknowledgement of different aspects of the personality, of which one is not always in full control, was considered proof of our primitiveness.

The Cassel culture so closely reflected that of the majority community and did not at any time truly challenge the external order of things. In true analytical style, it focused down, ever down, into the intrapsychic, often failing to acknowledge the fact that social pathology precedes psychopathology, and collective pathology precedes individual pathology. As Amos Wilson (1993: p. 68) acknowledged:

> This individualism tries to persuade us that this society is equal, and that this society makes available to all individuals equally the opportunity to advance in it, and if they fail, it is the result of their own personal problems. Of course, it becomes obvious that this kind of approach is a rationale and a rationalization by means of which the society itself ignores its own input as far as the failure of a person or people, such as our people, are concerned.

It helps us to ignore the impact of the social structures upon individual achievement and mobility. It tends almost literally to try and eradicate the ideas that the individual succeeds or fails within a social structure.

He goes on to say (p. 69):

This ideology speaks of such apparent neutral things as psychodynamic make-up of the individual; it speaks of weak egos; lack of personal integration, conflicts between Id, ego, and super-ego; the dark side of the personality overtaking the light side of the personality. All kinds of symptoms, names and intrapsychic mechanisms are invoked to explain the subjugation of some people and the domination of others; the so-called success of some and the failure of others.

For a black person to succeed at the Cassel Hospital was to fail as a black person because the culture of the Cassel is a microcosm of the society; yet, a much more in-depth experience could be had there, because it dealt with the realities of class, gender and group dynamics, and attempted at least to understand them. It still, however, required the black person to maintain his or her position in society, as the oppressed, in order for the status quo to be maintained and ignored, as evidenced by a colour blindness within the Cassel community as a whole. The treatment programme for patients, and the experience as a staff member, could help one to tinker around with the intrapsychic aspects, but never truly to challenge the social order of things, for example, white supremacy.

Armed with this experience, and an awareness of having worked in an analytical environment, where hidden agendas were exposed and personal pathology dissected, the lie within the truth became clear for me. This is what is important when working interculturally because, with the patient–therapist–nurse triad, there is a reality to the power–race dynamic.

No matter how pleasant, caring, understanding, intelligent, liberal or 'right on' Europeans are, the reality is that they are different. They hold an innate belief in their own abilities and power, which they are very prepared to share with you, as long as you do not threaten them in any meaningful way. When working with someone from a different race or culture, the bottom line with which one has to be engaged is the fear and anger that is generated once the equilibrium is challenged. The fact that, in my time at the Cassel, a large number of the therapists were either non-European or nonwhite truly means nothing. The nonwhite staff's ability to compensate for their nonwhiteness was profound. As Amos Wilson (1993: p. 36) said:

The individual who has amnesia suffers distortion of and blindness to reality. The individual who cuts himself off from his history is self-alienated. There's a whole part of himself that's completely shut off from his use. It's as if there were two parts. One part is unknown, yet because it is unknown doesn't mean that it is not effective. We have to devote energy to unknowing. We have to direct perception to unknowing. We have to say: Let me turn my face so I cannot see; let me not think about it. So the struggle to not know itself becomes creator of behaviour and personality structure. So the idea that not knowing one's history somehow permits one to escape it is a lie. In fact, it brings one under the domination of the more pernicious effects of that history and opens the personality up for self-alienation, self-destruction.

I do not recall any black male patient making it through the assessment phase of treatment. I believe that the failure of the Cassel as an inter-cultural arena was due to its true reflection of the community. How could this culture be dissecting the minutiae of things when not even able to discuss the blatantly obvious. It was not the treatment programme that failed as such, but that the wider community/society failed black people, and continues to do so.

Where the Cassel was different was that it acknowledged that it had a problem, but one that it could do nothing about because it could not change the way that a whole society viewed and used its power. It could only reflect it. Thus, helping people to understand their position within it, both intrapsychically and socially, enables them to understand what, within their personal experience and history, hinders them from fulfilling their potential. The Cassel is often accused of being rigid in its structure. New staff and patients buck against the system, furiously trying to make it bend and reshape it to fit their own need and personal pathology. The structural boundaries facilitate discussion of these requests, allowing both staff and patients to conceptualize the possible consequences of any proposed changes to: the individual, the nurse–patient relationship, the patient–therapist relationship, the nurse–therapist–patient relationship, the unit, the community and the hospital as a whole. By keeping the boundaries well defined, it is easier to see what the individual is doing within them, and to try to gain some understanding about why.

It was always a great pleasure to me that the Cassel had only three or four main rules. Everything else was strictly negotiable. The process of negotiation was eternal, creating a many-faceted depth of understanding.

The psychotherapeutic dynamics of black–white interactions

The dynamics of black–white interaction are a factor that I believe contributes towards the general paralysis experienced by most white staff in relation to black clients. White staff end up behaving ineffectually in their need to appear 'fair' and just, which is complicated by the fear of appearing to be, or being experienced by the black client to be, racist. They are either paralysed or overunderstanding. In fact, they are being racist, because they operate as if they do not expect the black client to have the capacity to deal with the challenge in whatever form it may take, or they are genuinely surprised when the black client does! As black staff, we do not want to work only with black clients, because this denies us the opportunity to show how much better we are at working interculturally. Clients, black or white, may not even countenance working with a black therapist, because they fear they will receive a substandard service. If we truly believe that everyone is equal, why are so many white people surprised when a black client is able to articulate his or her distress? On the other hand, I know that we all have to deal with racism, be it internalized or projected, but this becomes very difficult when people react as if you have called them a Nazi; once the issue of race is raised. There appears to be a fear that acknowledging racism automatically leads to fascism.

Europeans worked very hard to create a world order with themselves at the top, which happened to have facilitated a certain amount of fascism. The insistence on this world order is racist. It is, however, interesting to see how the Europeans can split themselves off from one another, but do not allow us to do the same. Not all white men are potential football hooligans, but all black men are potentially muggers or murderers. Could it be that the fear of a similar groupism being projected back helps to create the confusion between fascism and racism?

One has to deal with the reality that fascists use race as one of their criteria for oppression and/or annihilation, so, for one to deny the race issue displayed in colour blindness among staff and patients, even when families had mixed-race members, is an example of the fear of racism. The black component was never actively worked with or drawn attention to, although it was obviously felt at the Cassel. By focusing the work on intrapsychic analysis and on the exploration of community living (the work of the hospital), the problems of race, racism and oppression could be, and were, ignored. An area of mass discomfort and conflict was thus avoided.

Within the black community, ability is often projected on to the white people. For example, a black person generally does not apply for a job or a course unless a white person agrees it is a good idea. A piece of work is not validated unless it is approved by the white community. There remains a sense of being a fraud, a sense of self as like a house or pyramid of cards, which relies on others external to oneself, one's community, one's race, and to one's culture, not to rock the table on which the cards are placed. Wilson (1990: p. 65) wrote:

> The projective relations between the relatively powerful white community and the relatively powerless black community constitute an authentic process of transformed social interaction. The dominant white community, by controlling the rhythm of black community life, controls to a significant extent the setting and experience of black people, their self-perception and perception of reality. The dominant white community, by means of projection, acts in ways that organize the motivational systems of the black community so that those systems are functional reflections of the white community's psycho-political needs.

Did the Cassel Hospital culture, through its reflection of the wider community, unconsciously act out the exclusion of black people in the way that the community at large would like to do? Both parties are involved in joint projections. Both parties laid blame for the inability to have a successful outcome of treatment on the doorstep of the other. Both parties denied their emotional ambivalence towards each other. Nowadays, it is just not politically correct. Political correctness has an ability to create the same kind of paralysis. In dealing with racism, one has first to acknowledge its existence, not merely in a statement of intent or on equal opportunity policy, but more like the words through a stick of rock.

Our history is a major part of our cure. If we are not allowed to feel the feelings, express the pain, and understand and explore the dynamics between ourselves and the Europeans, no real therapeutic work can be done. There is no basis for a relationship and no possibility for true communication. Lenora Fulani (1988: p. 144), black American psychotherapist and politician, says in her essay, 'Women of colour do great therapy':

> All societies are in history even though our typical experience (both consciously and unconsciously) is a living only in society. For a feature of the society we live in is that it adapts people to society in a radically ahistoric fashion. Indeed, this adaptation to society is so complete that people often do not even have an awareness that they are in history. That history is something it is possible to adapt to. In our view (as social therapists) this deprivation of a sense of oneself as a historical entity is a major cause of all varieties of psychopathology.

Without history, we have no right to feel angry, hostile and confused, just as men have no justification for feeling humiliated by female bosses, or white people by black bosses. If we acknowledge our histories together and our societal conditioning, we would have a greater sense of sanity.

Development of the black psyche as a therapeutic tool

The Afrocentric perspective of intelligence envisions one wholistic (see Glossary), organized process. Thus, all political, artistic, economic, ethical and aesthetic issues are connected to the context of Afrocentric knowledge. Everything that you do, all that you are and will become, is intricately wrapped within the kente (see Glossary) of culture. Mind and matter, spirit and fact, truth and opinion, are all aspects of dimensions of one vital process (Asante, 1992: p. 38).

To free the black psyche from its enslavement to European ideology would be one of the most powerful world events, a powerful challenge to accepted world order, and hence a serious political issue. Imagine a notion of divinity (spirit) running through each and every one of us and each and every thing, to be able to trust one's instincts and run with it, with the ego put to one side. A selflessness that was once our undoing would now be our salvation. Non-Europeans have tried consistently for several hundred years to follow the European lead. The inability to have a wholistic approach, to acknowledge the cosmology of things, the blueprint of the universe, and human beings' place within it. To see and feel the truth, rather than to intellectualize, and hear only what is said, and to know because you know. To be able to value your insperience (see Glossary), as much as you have been taught to value experience. We are more than a darkened version of white people. We are an entity in our own right. We need to reclaim the primitive and the natural.

Recently, I became aware of how unobtainable the Eurocentric notions of perfection were; for example, a European concept of beauty, which is blonde, blue-eyed, and virtually anorexic. A pure voice is a pubescent male, or is operatically trained so that it sounds more like an instrument than a human, not natural, not in the order of things, not something that can be developed, mastered and improved naturally.

There is a youth culture. We follow people who know nothing of life, just because they are young and, as part of their developmental process, need change. Afrocentric beauty glorifies the most common of features, and the most practical ones that enhance your purpose within this incarnation.

To be 'strong', current black slang for a beautiful girl, is that she is fit or has a healthy body. A beautiful voice is deep, resonant, rhythmic and matured. A culture is that which reveres and respects its old for the experience and knowledge they have gained. Does it not make more sense? We truly have to recapture the notion of primitive, in the same way that we reclaimed the word 'black'. There is a need to look to the old and learn rather than hanker for the new. Black students' basic psychological learning must include: Niam Akbar (1985), Wade Nobles (1992), Amos Wilson (1990), Francis Cress-Wesley (1992) and others, who present different aspects of psychological thinking and developmental frameworks and thought to balance and rival any of the well-taught European schools of psychology. We must acknowledge the developments and processes in thinking that resulted in their radical psychologist and psychiatrist labels. The only thing that was radical about them was that they put themselves, our selves, our black selves, in the centre of the enquiry and exploration.

We, as black people, must familiarize ourselves with the works of our people, the methods and treatment modes that have been developed for us, and by us, so that we are as familiar with them as we are with the European ones. Basic knowledge and skills are being lost with each generation; for example, nutritional and herbal medicine, and the significance and power of colours, gems and crystal. The new ideas are not being made accessible through the European education systems. What works for white folk does not necessarily work for us. We need to do more than talk secretly and shamefully about how different we are from Europeans and start to glory in that difference. We must begin the work to reclaim our consciousness.

Psychosocial care within the black community

The Cassel Hospital is often disparaged within the black community because it works in such a privileged environment, with staff and client groups also considered to be highly privileged; whereas, in reality, many of the families are working class, of mixed race, and are often lone parents. This reality does nothing to dispel the myth. There is a belief within the psychiatric establishment that no real work is being done unless one is on the front line in a multidisciplinary, multicultural, inner-city, deprived area, with a high nonwhite clientele, which is struggling against incredible odds and increasingly dealing with symptom control.

The Cassel offers treatment in a respectful manner, acknowledging that there is not a magic wand or wand waver; there is no easy solution to treatment. Rather, the treatment takes time to uproot the causes of difficulties before adaptation can be made and internalized. It is true that the Cassel does not provide the kind of care that is offered in other environments. It is not, and can never be, an active arm of social control, and, as such, it is an excellent model for residential projects, for, like the Cassel, these should be based on integrity.

No successful treatment programme can be developed for the black community that does not incorporate the psychological, the social, the physical, and the political. These realities have to be woven into any treatment plan. We cannot concentrate solely on the individual's psychic state. The plan must incorporate within it an acknowledgement of and working with the societal position of black people. As therapists, we must stop the political lie and modelling it as the norm. We have internalized a system and it has become a part of our confusion and our disorientation.

Both intercultural and 'black on black' psychotherapy help as a key to increase the ability for self-acceptance, self-love and trusting one's own instincts, one's blackness. Both these forms of therapy incorporate the issue of race as central to any intrapychic work, practised and taught at Nafsiyat and Shanti (see Organizations). The black on black therapy model that we are developing in this country is based on the integration of integrative psychotherapy with social political and racial and spiritual realities (Ipamo and Black Therapy Association, see Organizations). Integration and acceptance of ourselves within the black community is essential before any work can be done across cultures.

Group work/therapy helps to minimize the sense of isolation that the majority of black people feel, and helps to undo the damage created by our separation from each other and from our past. This work cannot be done effectively in a mixed community. We have no time for dealing with the oppression hierarchy, or for explaining what we have to do, and why. Work with black people needs to begin during education and in an understanding of the fallacy of white social order as part of their normal lives. Otherwise, the work needs to be in alternative establishments created specifically for black people as specialties, not just when it is all too late, when they enter the institutions designed to meet the needs of others. We need to incorporate within our lives the sense of community, family, and true religion: the remembering of all aspects of our being, redefining our own psychology, our own spirit, our own selves and our own God, so that we will not be found wanting and will have prepared the way for our children. Maat (in keeping with divine law).

References

Akbar, N. (1985). *The Community of Self*, (revised). MIND.
Asante, M.K.K. (1992). *Afrocentricity and Knowledge*. African World Press.
Cress-Wesley, F. (1992). *The Isis Papers*. Third World Press.
Fulani, L. (1988). *The Psychology of Everyday Racism and Sexism*. Harrington Press.
Nobles, W. (1992). *Standing by the River*. Kara Press and Kemetic Book Club.
Wilson, A.N. (1990). *Black on Black Violence*. Afrikan World Infosystems.
Wilson, A.N. (1993). *The Falsification of African Consciousness*. Afrikan World Infosystems.

Glossary

insperience – initiate information, receive insight for one's indwelling intelligence.

kente – from the Shanti language, which is spoken in Ghana. There are many interpretations of the word, the definition I am using means creative diversity. It has also been used to describe the evolution of ideas, that all good ideas must come to an end, as portrayed in the Indwelling Intelligence Museum of Ghana.

kente – African multipatterned, multicoloured interwoven traditional cloth.

wholistic – not secretive.

Organizations

Black Therapy Association (runs Black Therapy Diploma course and Black therapy journal), c/o 15 Harpenden Road, London SE27 0AG.

Ipamo (Black Mental Health Service, alternative to hospital), c/o 332 Brixton Road, London SW9 7AA.

Nafsiyat (Intercultural Psychotherapy Centre), 278 Seven Sisters Road, Finsbury Park, London N4 2HY.

Shanti (Intercultural Women's Psychotherapy Service), 1a Dalbury House, Ferndale Road, Brixton, London SW9 8AP.

Chapter 16
Learning through experience

Louise de Lambert

Socrates described the unexamined life as the life not worth living. My theme is concerned with the value of examining the working life of nurses, particularly their relationships with patients. This examination can happen more readily with willingness and courage when there is a 'culture of enquiry' (Main, 1989) which supports this process. Such exploration requires not only legitimacy but also security, which is provided by clear working structures, defined professional roles and regular meetings in which the events, uncertainties and strains of work can be shared, studied and contained.

The Cassel Hospital has a psychoanalytical orientation, so it follows that legitimate examination concerns not only conscious but also unconscious matters. The understanding of hidden feelings and conflicts underlies this work. In this therapeutic community, opportunities to discover new ways of working are constantly available.

Joinings and leavings are important. Who does not remember the day they started school or the day they left home? At the Cassel Hospital, this is acknowledged in the careful way that new staff and patients are introduced to the hospital community. I will describe my own experience of joining the nursing staff to illustrate this.

Orientation

The first week at the hospital was shared with the colleague who had started with me. A very full and well-planned introductory programme was arranged for us, so that we could meet everyone in the hospital, from consultants to cleaners. The pattern of these meetings helped us to understand the working relationships and responsibilities which were so important to the functioning of the hospital. This was tested by our having to produce a diagram at the end of the week, illustrating the staffing structure, showing who was responsible for what to whom, and what role relationships were involved in each person's work.

At the end of each day of the first week, we met for half an hour with Matron to discuss our day. We were invited to reflect on our experiences and feelings, and to talk about them, especially our newness, and our needs and anxieties. What a powerful experience it is to be listened to, taken seriously, treated with interest and respect! After this first week, we were introduced to other elements of our work and learning. The care, attention and thoughtfulness, lavished – as it felt – on us as new nurses, and the evident planning and preparation for our arrival, helped with the inevitable anxieties of being new.

This experience and the encouraged reflection on it began my awakening to the importance of beginnings and attachment. We were shown the films of Robertson and Robertson (1953) and joined in discussion about the effects of separation on infants and young children, and on the important work of John Bowlby (1951) on attachment and loss.

Learning on the families unit

The families unit was where we began our work with patients. I was in the care of a senior nurse who was guide, mentor and teacher; together we went on my first home visit to a family before they were to be admitted. The aim was to help this distressed and troubled family to take the steps from home to our hospital and also to prepare for their arrival with other patients in the unit. My own very recent newness was relevant and I was encouraged to draw on this experience in introducing the family into hospital.

At the same time, we began our tutorials on human development which were to continue throughout the year. In reading and discussing how a mother and family prepare for a new baby, another aspect of new beginnings was brought into awareness. Associated with these tutorials were observation visits to the hospital's nursery school, which catered for two-to-five-year-old children from the hospital and the local community. Our first focus was to observe the leaving and joinings of the children as they were brought to the nursery and collected at the end of each session. We observed especially the parent–child relationship: the goodbyes and greetings, how the child responded to these and how they varied among the different parents and children.

Some weeks later, the senior nurse of the families unit, and also our tutor in human development studies, went on a short holiday. At our first tutorial after her return, one of the nurses launched into a bitter complaint about her, criticizing her failure to attend to some roster detail. So sharp and reproachful were her words that the senior nurse was in tears. I was embarrassed and alarmed, until she, through her tears, talked with us about a child's often antagonistic response to reunion with his or her mother after a separation, which we had seen recently illustrated in the Robertson films. This dramatic on-the-spot connection of infant and adult to the distress of both nurses, gave it new meaning. My dismay subsided, understanding dawned, and the impact of this remained and was the first of many demonstrations of psychoanalytical sense. There was no rebuke, no counterattack, but a thought-provoking, deep and helpful understanding. This culture of enquiry was not a culture of criticism; understanding, not judgement, was important.

Our work on the unit was to be involved, alongside patients, in the running of the domestic life of the place, the care of the children, and participation in the wider hospital life.

Nursing is a strange trade, in which mundane and ordinary concerns and activities are mixed with awareness and responsibility for matters of acute significance. Experiences, such as suicidal despair, self-starvation, violent impulses, bewilderment and withdrawal from others, start to be contained and managed by patients and nurses as they deal with the business of getting up in the morning, managing meals, household tasks, conversation and many other demands and opportunities of daily living. The closeness, immediacy and apparent ordinariness of the nurse's work with patients engages the nurse's natural unguarded self. Much of nursing work is intuitive or responsive. The recognition and valuing of responses and feelings enable nurses to use them for better understanding of interactions and relationships. The therapeutic relevance of nursing is often manifested within the seemingly ordinary experience of getting together with patients over shared activities. This is the base for the nurse–patient relationship, once rather overlooked, now much more recognized as a crucial element in nursing work and its effectiveness.

The necessary opportunities for reflection, analysis and understanding are provided in the many meetings which form such an important part of the therapeutic community structure. These include frequent meetings of nursing staff, daily multidisciplinary staff meetings and various training seminars. There is a balance to be found between the defensive avoidance afforded by many meetings and the strain and difficulties which can accrue from intensive and demanding involvement without the helpful sharing and discussion with colleagues.

While the clinical work of the Cassel Hospital is specialized and richly enhanced by the training and experience of senior staff, many of its methods, particularly the seminar training, may be successfully transplanted into other settings.

Learning in seminars

The seminar setting can quite successfully include people with a wide range of experience, namely, newly qualified and senior nurses. Regular meetings of a group of six to ten works well. Ninety minutes is a satisfactory time for this when the group meets often. In situations where this is not possible, weekend seminars offer an intensive period of work. The group has a leader or convenor with a special responsibility, which includes helping the group to keep to the task of studying the nurse–patient relationship, with emphasis on the nurse's experience, responses and feelings. There is always the opportunity to share a nursing problem or issue in whatever form. To have a problem that can be felt, described and shared is an achievement which makes a useful beginning.

When I now supervise or lead a seminar, I do not ask people to come with a well-prepared case, but like to hear whatever comes up at the time. It is usually something of immediate concern and importance. Colleagues within the group contribute not only their ideas about the presentation, but also to the atmosphere generated within the group, from which there is information to be gained about the nurse's story. For example, the level of interest, compassion, laughter or boredom can be important factors in understanding what is going on. The group's capacity for attunement to the feelings evoked in the nurse by her patient will be enhanced by the members' own experience of being heard and understood themselves and the collective wisdom developed over time within the group. Learning to talk about emotional responses to patients can be difficult and takes time to develop. It concerns observing and discussing one's own self, noticing the irritations, fondness or confusion that the nurse may feel for a particular person, and having the courage to name the feelings. It is difficult to be really honest about some of these feelings and to trust other group members enough to reveal and explore them. Conflicts or disagreements with patients and colleagues are important aspects to discuss.

One of the best ways to hear about a clinical problem is for the nurse to describe a recent event or to give an example of a characteristic situation for which help is sought. Some examples are given below of seminar work with different groups of nurses at the Cassel Hospital and, more recently, in New Zealand.

Karen's story

In a group of nurses working in the psychiatric ward of a children's hospital, Karen told us of a series of uncomfortable conversations with the mother of 14-year-old Cindy, in which she had felt trapped. The mother, Margaret, was very critical of Karen's care of Cindy and found fault in many matters. She blamed the nurse for the loss of Cindy's sweatshirt, criticized the hospital diet as totally unsuitable for her daughter's acne, and demanded more information about the unit's treatment programme. Karen was hurt and indignant, found herself justifying the therapeutic plans and trying to convince Margaret of how much she had done for Cindy.

I noticed the similarity in the way she sought to convince us in the group of Karen's special efforts, although her colleagues were in no doubt about her commitment. They knew she had stayed on late to go with Cindy to the shops in search of a special skin care lotion she wanted and Karen was known for being conscientious. Perhaps she had been too conscientious. We wondered what other feelings may have been hidden in Margaret's complaints, whether she might have felt inadequate, critical of herself and perhaps bewildered, and hurt by the fact that, while Cindy had settled in well to the unit, there were terrible rows when she went home for weekends. Margaret had confided to one of the nurses in the group that she did not want Cindy at home again, ever. This was more painful, more real, and allowed compassion for mother and daughter in their struggles. Four weeks later, Karen reported back at the next group meeting, saying that, interestingly, there had been a good talk between her and Margaret, who had said how jealous she felt of Karen's friendly relationship with Cindy and the success that the unit was having with her. What different possibilities there were now. We guessed that something had changed and that Margaret maybe now had some sense of Karen's readiness to listen to her.

It is remarkable how often this sort of discussion in a group is followed by changes and nurses reporting new developments.

There is a great deal of important contact between these nurses and the parents of the children, some of whom are very disturbed and difficult to manage. The nurses are often the target of attack, criticism and dissatisfaction. This discussion had relevance for many in the group. It can be helpful to understand that the dreaded visit of a critical, raging parent may both conceal and express feelings of guilt and failure.

Ann's problem

Ann was working as a nursing assistant on placement in a therapeutic community as part of her social work training. Rather hesitantly, she brought her dilemma of working with Richard, a formidably clever man who had worked for a publishing firm before his admission.

In the hospital he seemed very friendly with some of the patients who had formed an 'in' group. Ann found him critical and disparaging of her. She felt small and inadequate; in fact he was over six feet tall and she was a slim five feet two inches. They were both members of a creative writing group in the hospital. On behalf of this group, Richard had invited a local author to come and discuss his work. Ann had let him know when she, as the nurse involved with this community activity, would be available. Her problem, as she brought it to the seminar, was that Richard had made the arrangement for the one evening she could not be there. She was afraid to take a stand with Richard and she did not know what to do. Ann had described her predicament well; many nurses in the seminar could empathize with her. We reflected on the fact that she was relatively young, new to the staff, and not a registered nurse. It was interesting that she should be the victim of Richard's exclusion and intimidation. Many of the nurses and patients were wary of him and kept away from close encounters. When we looked carefully, we could not find anyone he was really close to, within the hospital or beyond. By using the concept of projection (the defence in which disavowed aspects of the self are attributed to another), we formed a hypothesis that Ann's uncomfortable feelings of insignificance and uncertainty might give us a clue to what lay unconsciously behind Richard's superior and disdainful attitude to others. There was thoughtful support for Ann to tackle the problem bravely, to protest at being ignored and insist on being included according to the original arrangements of the writing group. If she yielded to the temptation to agree with Richard that she did not matter, that it was just a mistake, and that she was being awkward and annoying to pursue it, important opportunities would have been missed. With anger and resistance, Richard had to face what he had done, and Ann's feelings. It helped him to come nearer to his own fear of being overlooked and excluded, and his bullying defence against feeling insignificant.

Soon after this, a slump into depression enabled him to work with his therapist about his guilt and feelings of alienation and worthlessness.

Ann learnt significantly about valuing herself, her feelings and observations, and about not backing off from difficult encounters. In using her feelings to understand, not allowing them to keep her excluded, she was also offering Richard a model of relating to others which could integrate and express vulnerable feelings. With the working relationship maintained she could be alongside him when he was miserable, and, rarely for him, he had not this time effectively pushed someone away, with the usual resulting isolation. At the next seminar, we were interested to hear how she had used the work we had done and she felt supported and pleased about how well she had responded.

Support for Elizabeth

At a monthly meeting with nurses working in the psychiatric ward of a children's hospital, the discussion began with an account of an argument between the nurses and management. They were indignant that one of their team had been sent to look after a seriously undernourished girl who had been transferred for physical care to one of the other wards for the weekend because she was too ill to go home as most of the children did. Elizabeth, the nurse on whose behalf the indignation and protest was being expressed, was in the group. I asked her how it had been for her to go to the other ward to nurse this patient. She spoke very movingly about her experience, of the terrible thinness of this young girl, Janine, who had a nasogastric tube through which she was being fed against her will. Elizabeth talked of sitting with Janine, about her acute misery and her wish to die. She said she felt the anorexia had her 'by the throat', and she felt utterly hopeless. Elizabeth seemed unperturbed at first, but she described her very difficult experience. She, as well as the rest of us, felt the impact of it. The whole of her shift had been spent exclusively with this very unhappy and troubling patient. The group was able to see how their outrage and argument had got in the way of perceiving their colleague's pain, and of offering any support or sharing of the task. When we reflected on it, there was a chance to see that the burden of this shift of special nursing was too much for one person.

With the opportunity to describe her experience in some detail, Elizabeth was tearful and more in touch with her distress. She had been very painfully aware of the patient's intense unhappiness and her moving account helped the rest of the group to appreciate it more poignantly. There had been a tendency to respond only with exasperation and frustration to Janine, who was so difficult to care for and who frightened people with the severity of her starvation.

When distress can be talked about, shared, known by others and understood, it is more manageable and less likely to be held for too long.

If indignation and outrage only had prevailed, these developments may not have happened. The seminar leader's separateness from the group helped, as well as her interest in enquiring about what might be concealed behind the initial communication and complaint. It became more complicated as we grappled with the difficulties of dealing with the mixed feelings towards this patient of anger, concern and uselessness.

The outcome for nurse management was new thinking about the roster for this kind of intensive individual nursing.

The prospects for Janine were good in the long term and an important factor was the nursing staff's capacity to hold both pain in the present and hope for the future for the family and the patient through a very difficult year.

Individual attention in a group setting

The next example is from a psychiatric hospital functioning as a therapeutic community. The conflict between attending to distressed individuals and being available in a group setting is a familiar one for psychiatric nurses, and the frightening escalation of self-harming behaviour is a conern often brought to group seminars.

At the seminar, a nurse, Lynette, told us about a young woman, Hilary, who had been in the hospital for some time. As an only child, Hilary had experienced difficulty in leaving home and her attempts at various jobs had failed as she succumbed to minor illnesses and loss of confidence. She had few friends and felt anxious in social settings. Her admission had followed a series of attempts to harm herself by cutting her wrists and taking overdoses of analgesics. She had formed a strong attachment to Lynette, her primary nurse. Lynette had been on evening duty, with responsibility for nursing all the patients in the ward. As she arrived on duty, Hilary had been waiting for her at the front door, a forlorn figure in her droopy cardigan with an urgent and tearful request for Lynette to spend time with her in her room for some private conversation and special attention. This was a familiar sort of situation, not only for Lynette. Many others in the seminar had the experience of feeling torn between the plea for personal attention or 'individual time', as it was called by patients, and the responsibilities and activities in the ward with the other patients. Some nurses felt much more important and valuable in this sort of one-to-one relationship, involved in an individual's pain and problems. Lynette recalled feeling both flattered and put upon, but irritated that she had not even taken off her coat or met her colleagues before being claimed by Hilary's demand on her.

This very familiar quandary for nurses in a therapeutic community had been discussed on other occasions when we had identified the conflict between a patient's wish for a response to her illness and incapacity and a nurse's aim to encourage healthy functioning and social activities. For Hilary, the nursing aims, which she had participated in designing, were to help her to become more independent and capable, and less self-absorbed, and to develop skills which might support her ambition of doing teacher training. She and her therapist were working to explore and understand her hostile dependence and failure to separate successfully from her family.

Lynette responded to the request by suggesting that Hilary should go with her to the social committee meeting she wanted to attend. The patient refused and renewed her distressed demands with some threatening undertones. Lynette acknowledged the urgency of the need Hilary felt, but restated her own responsibility to be at the meeting and the invitation for Hilary to go with her. After standing firm, feeling guilty, anxious and irritated, Lynette went to the meeting and, within a few minutes, was joined there by Hilary, wrists intact, a bit grumpy, but able to participate quite well. Lynette was warm in her acknowledgement of the choice Hilary had made. She then had the chance, however reluctantly, to join with others in planning an outing.

Someone asked Lynette how she had managed to do it differently this time. We had heard in previous meetings of her tendency to become caught up in individual sessions instead of being 'around'. Lynette talked of her anxiety about Hilary 'doing something awful', how controlled she felt by such threats, and also of her irritation with Hilary and her very clear wish to do a different sort of nursing on this evening.

Earlier in the week, a case conference about Hilary had registered concern about her lack of progress; if anything, she seemed to have become more dependent and there was a suggestion that admission to hospital had been a mistake. The original good nursing care plans had in reality been sabotaged and put aside. In the nurses' meeting, there had been a rallying of support for consistency and challenge to help Hilary make progress. It seemed that Lynette had been informed and challenged by previous seminar discussions, the clinical conference and her growing understanding of psychosocial nursing. We had looked at how the admission to hospital can be experienced by a patient as a longed-for opportunity to be looked after, which can invite regression and then hostility when the demands and challenges of the community are experienced. For Hilary, what happened in hospital was becoming very like the situation at home, in which she had felt so restricted and disturbed. For Lynette, the challenge was to develop her skills in group-based nursing, to be less controlled by anxieties and claims for special attention, and to take some risks with the support and understanding of colleagues.

The role of the seminar leader

The role of the seminar leader is to provide structure and focus for the group and assist the process of exploration and understanding. The capacity for this is helped by the leader's own learning experiences. The examples I have used in this account are drawn from my own collection of stories, which seems to be the way my learning is registered, remembered and available to me.

Lynette's experience recalled an event during my first year at the Cassel. At a Monday community meeting, Andrea, who had spent a miserable weekend in bed feeling depressed, made a public complaint about my neglect of her emotional needs and distress. I had done the long weekend shift and based my community-centred nursing in the sewing room, where quite a large group of us had congregated. While I completed a dress, someone else cut out a pattern and we helped another put in a zip. Although I had made regular visits to Andrea's bedside and she had been invited to join us, I found myself guiltily anticipating a reprimand. After all, I was a well-trained hospital nurse! After hearing the account of the weekend, Matron, from across the room, said that sewing was just the sort of activity she expected nurses to be involved in and she was sorry that Andrea had not been able to enjoy the weekend. My relief and this support helped me to integrate the growing notions I had of psychosocial nursing and the conflicting obligation I felt to attend the individual's needs at the bedside. The experience of not being reprimanded, and being expected and trusted to make my own decisions, happened often and helpfully during my training.

One of the important opportunities in a seminar is for the sharing of uncertainty or discomfort. It takes some courage and trust to expose one's work for scrutiny and this deserves respect. New understanding and learning is quite often achieved in a context of anxiety or distress. Difficulties push us towards looking for help, new ideas, or some way of changing things that are unsatisfactory. Uncomfortable learning can be significant and lasting. While theoretical ideas are useful and contribute significantly to some skills and understanding, there is a dimension of learning which is gained only through experience.

Empathy, compassion and emotional understanding develop through the direct experience of those qualities in another, perhaps a parent, mentor or teacher. The people most likely to recognize their colleagues' distress are those who have already had the experience of their own distress being responded to and recognized. This particular form of learning through experiences develops qualities of sensitivity and responsiveness.

A colleague was travelling in a train which killed a man who had deliberately thrown himself in front of it. She returned to the hospital where she worked and recounted this experience over afternoon tea to several people who said, 'How awful,' and passed on. Eventually, this was responded to by one who heard rather differently and, with im- mediate concern for more than the words, said, 'You have just witnessed a death. I think you'd better come and talk about it.' Then, with a colleague who was empathic and emotionally available and who recognized her trauma, she could cry over the shock of her experience and share the ghastly images she had of the body under the carriage in which she had been. Her fear and distress were acknowledged and seen as legitimate and understandable.

Some time after the incident of the suicide on the railway line, that nurse was convening a seminar group. A story which had been around the hospital all day was told yet again by Jenny, the night nurse, who had stayed on duty to come to the seminar. Late on the night before, she had been telephoned by an anonymous male caller telling her that a bomb had been planted in the hospital and, unless she agreed to participate in a sexually provocative conversation, he would not tell her where it was. At the time, bomb hoaxes were commonplace and such 'nuisance' telephone calls were not unusual, but the nurse was alone and felt abused and terrified by this encounter, yet felt it would be ridiculous to make a fuss about it. Clearly, Jenny was troubled enough to stay on for the group seminar, which would be another chance to share her experience. The seminar leader had herself experienced the benefit of being listened to in the way just described, which heard and acknowledged her own emotional responses to a nasty and frightening event. She was, therefore, able to hear this story and allow it to have the impact and significance it deserved. Being heard and responded to allowed the nurse finally to realize for herself the full horror of her experience and to weep about it and recover from her fear and upset. In this, she had an important learning experience, which would enhance her own capacity to respond sensitively to others' distress.

This is an example of that dimension of learning through experience which is about having the emotional aspects of distress recognized accurately and responded to in a way that reaches the inner vulnerable feelings. Such experiences bring about significant changes within the self. One of the most important principles at the Cassel Hospital is that containment, understanding and professional development of the staff is of paramount importance. If the feelings of workers are taken seriously and they are well looked after, this will be reflected in the quality of patient care. People tend to do to others as they have been done to themselves. This is particularly important in management, training and clinical work. The most effective way of helping nurses to develop relationship skills, understanding, good communication and professional strength, is to ensure that they encounter the same skills in their relationships with their colleagues, teachers and managers.

The ability to face distress, acknowledge and share feelings, and learn through the process of understanding the examined experience, makes the professional working life infinitely more valuable.

References

Bowlby, J. (1951). *Maternal Care and Mental Health*. World Health Organization.
Main, T.F. (1989). The concept of the therapeutic community: variations and vicissitudes. In *The Ailment and Other Psychoanalytic Essays* (J. Johns, ed.) pp. 123–141, Free Association Books.
Robertson, J. and Robertson, J. (1953). *Young Children in Brief Separation series: John, Jane, Kate, Thomas, Lucy* (Films and videos). Concord Video and Film Council, Ipswich.

Index

Abuse *see* Childhood sexual abuse
Access to Personal Files Act 1987, 96
Accountability, 189, 194–6
Action research, 19–21
  enhancement approach, 20
Activities, patients'
  Austen Riggs Center, 57
  bicycle maintenance, 77
  clinical context, 73–4
  cycles in, 80
  definition, 73
  emergence of self, 77–81
  encouraging self-esteem, 77–8
  patient involvement, 74–6
  physical activities, 76
  play component of, 78
  poetry reading, 76–7
  role changes during, 78–9
  social purpose, 73–4, 76–7, 81
  therapeutic purpose, 73–4, 76–7, 81
  types of, 73
  and voluntary space, 79–81
  and work, blurring of boundaries, 80
Adult learning, 164–5

Anorexic patient, seminar case example, 216–17
Association for Psychoanalytic Psychotherapy, 17
Association of Psychosexual Nurses, 160
Assumption of no order, 101, 104
Attitudes in psychosocial nursing *see* Knowledge, skills and attitudes
Austen Riggs Center, 53–4
  nurse–doctor relationship, 57–8
  nurse exchange programme, 56–8
  nurses' role, 54–5
  patients' activities, 57
  seminar training, 55
Authority
  appropriate use of, 194–6
  example, 195–6
  hatred of authority figures, 86–7, 92
Autonomy paradigm, 34

Balint-style seminars, 153
  case example, 170–2
  mental health placements, 167

Balint-style seminars – *continued*
  working with older people,
    181–6
Balint-style seminars, research
    study
  findings, 172–3
  group characteristics, 167–8
  group discussion themes, 168
  group discussions, 169–72
  methodology, 167–8
  teacher's role in discussion,
    174–5
Behaviour, disturbed, type of, 72
Bicycle maintenance, 77
Biographical work with older
    people, 178–87
  authentic picture of older
    people, 179
  examples from Balint-style
    seminars, 181–6
  recurring patterns, 180
  therapeutic review of life,
    179–80
Black community, psychosocial
    care in, 207–8
Black Mental Health Service
    (Ipamo), 208, 209
'Black on black' psychotherapy,
    208
Black psyche, as a therapeutic tool,
    206–7
Black Therapy Association, 208,
    209
Black–white interactions, 203–5
Blackness
  and the Cassel Hospital,
    198–200, 201, 201–2, 203
  European, a dilemma, 200–3
Body memories
  an accident-prone child, 122–4

body and memory refusing to
    die, 128–30
  a child overwhelmed, 124–8
  impetus to seek help, 129–30
  as painful protection, 123–4
  and self-destruction, 130–2
Body tissues, containing pain, 121
Boundaries, 24

Care-workers, definition, xv
  Case conferences, 193
Cassel Hospital
  address, xvii
  and blackness, 198–200, 201,
    201–2, 203
  culture of enquiry, 7, 13, 24
  current practice, 9–10
  history, 5–6
  learning in seminars, 213–17
  learning on the families unit,
    211–13
  middle-classness of, 199–200
  nurse induction programme,
    210–11
  nursery school, 211–12
  patients, 6
  psychosocial nurse training, 46–7
  psychosocial nursing
    development, 6, 8–9
  regular meetings, 10
  responding to nurses' distress,
    221
  therapeutic community
    principles, 7–8
  treatment aspects, 6–7
Cassel Hospital research study
  analysis, 22–33
  research design, 19–21
  research methodology, 21–2
  workshops, 21–2

Cassel Hospital Strategy for
    Nursing Group, 11–12
Cassel model
    abstract and practical levels, 11
    ongoing questioning of ideas, 13
    pressures dictating need for, 12
    rationale for, 11–14
    see also Psychosocial model of
        practice
Change
    by exception, 55
    incremental, 55–6
    influences on, 58
    paradigm change, 56
    pendulum, 56
    resistance to, 58
    types of, 55–6
Child and family consultation
    service, case study
    active participation with
        families, 108
    assessment visits, 111–12
    coping with illness and
        treatment, 114–17
    early changes, 113–14
    fears of bone marrow
        transplant, 117
    initial interview, 110–11
    nurse–patient relationship, 113,
        117
    nursing aim, 112–13
    referral, 109–10
    scapegoating, 109–10
Child care legislation and policy
    guidelines, 96
Child protection, 95–6
    assumption of no order, 101, 104
    bureaucracy and abuse
        minimization, 97
    case study, 102–7

changes by families, 101–2
comprehensive assessments, 99
containment, 100–1
hold and support function, 100
parental construct, 99
practitioners' self-protective
    systems, 97–9
responsibility within, 98–9
staff support, 97
training courses, 97–8
Child Protection Register, 95–6
Childhood sexual abuse, adult
        survivor of, case study
    approaching discharge, 91–2
    assessment meeting, 88
    background, 83–4
    and eating disorders, 86
    family meetings with husband,
        90–1
    hatred of authority figures, 86–7,
        92
    inpatient assessment, 85–7
    laxative abuse, 88–9
    lessons learnt, 92
    nightmares, 89
    nursing, 88–90
    outpatient assessment, 84–5
    physical symptoms, 84, 87, 92
    preadmission home visit, 84–5
    support for nurse, 89, 93
Children Act 1989, 96, 98, 101
Civil servants, 59–60
Clinical supervision, 32, 188–97
    and accountability, 189, 194–6
    to combat errors and
        shortcomings, 189–90
    concept of, 190
    difficult professional
        relationships, 195–6
    and giving of self, 190

Clinical supervision – *continued*
  as help with emotional stress,
    190–2, 192–3
  holding in, 190
  and support, 190–2
  welcomed by nurses, 188–9
Common sense, 59
Computerization, example of
  wasted resources, 48–50
Containment, 103
  of distress or feelings, 51, 105,
    107
  to perform a task, 79
  setting, 84
Co-operative enquiry, 20
Counselling
  experience of feeling
    understood, 153
  psychosexual, 159–60
Criticism from patient's relative,
  seminar case example, 214–15
Culture of enquiry, 7, 13, 24, 210,
  212
  institutional, 46

Demanding patient, seminar case
  examples, 183–4, 186, 217–19
Dependency, 28
  seminar case example, 181–2,
    184–5
Diploma in Psychosocial Nursing, 9
Diploma in Sexual Health Care,
  160
Direct observation, 42, 44
  see also Ethnography
Discourse, 60
  see also Words

Eating disorders, and childhood
  sexual abuse, 86

Education and training
  adult learning, 164–5
  Black Therapy Diploma course,
    209
  Diploma in Psychosocial
    Nursing, 9
  Diploma in Sexual Health Care,
    160
  ENB 660 course in
    psychodynamic ideas, 17
  ENB 985 Principles of
    Psychosexual Counselling for
    Nurses, 159
  ENB course, Nursing Elderly
    People, 178
  experiential learning, 46–7,
    165–6, 210–21
  by intercolleague meetings, 46–7
  nurse induction programme,
    210–11
  psychosocial nursing, 8–9, 46–7
  RCN courses, 17
  seminar training, 55
  social workers, 97–8, 101
  theory–practice gap, 164
  see also Learning; Psychosexual
    nursing seminars; Seminars
Ego-strength, 79–80
Elderly *see* Biographical work with
  older people; Older people
Emotional
  damage, 51
  distress, 42
  holding, 44, 50
  neglect, 95, 102, 104
  response for understanding, 44
Emotions
  emotional damage, 70
  emotional domain, 76
  emotional expectations, 72

emotional holding, 44, 50
emotional neglect, 95, 102, 104
emotional reaction, 42, 43
emotional response, 44, 213
emotional work of nurses, 45–6
learning from, 43
logic and, 44
mind-body interplay, 124
nurses' reactions to, 42
poetry and, 77
v. logic, 43–7, 49–50
English National Board (ENB)
courses
ENB 660 in psychodynamic
ideas, 17
ENB 985 Principles of
Psychosexual Counselling for
Nurses, 159
Nursing Elderly People, 178
Enhancement approach, in action
research, 20
Enquiry, culture of *see* Culture of
enquiry
Environment, in psychosocial
model of practice, 24–5
Ethnography (participant
observation), 44, 45, 46, 51
example, 47–9
see also Direct observation
Experiential learning, 46–7, 165–6,
210–21

Failures, usefulness of, 27, 42–3
Family
case studies, 102, 108
losses, 6
meeting, 90
person and, 34
survival after abuse, 119
working relationship with, 95

Families' unit, learning on,
211–13
Fawcett's metaparadigms, 22–3,
33–4
Feelings
and behaviour, 73
denied, 113
hidden, 214
naming', 213
nurses', 155, 157, 191, 195, 215
patients', 72, 158, 161
shame, 75
students', 156, 161
thinking about, 171, 172
Frameworks *see* Nursing models

Goals and outcomes of
psychosocial nursing
environment, 24–5
health, 28–9
nursing, 30–2
person, 26–7
'Good enough' parenting, 96
Government policy guidelines
child care, 96, 98
NHS reforms, 60–1
Group therapy, 5–6

Health, in psychosocial model of
practice, 28–9
Helplessness, in external trauma,
125
Holding, in clinical supervision,
190

Impotence, seminar case example,
156
Insperience, 206, 209
Institute of Psychosexual Medicine,
153, 160

Integrity, injuries to, 129–30
Intercultural psychotherapy, 208
Intercultural Psychotherapy Centre
    (Nafsiyat), 208, 209
Intercultural Women's
    Psychotherapy Service
    (Shanti), 209
Intervention model, 72–3
    see also Activities
Intimidation from patient, seminar
    case example, 215–16
Involvement with patients see
    Nurse–patient relationship
Ipamo (Black Mental Health
    Service), 208, 209

Kente, 206, 209
Knowledge, skills and attitudes in
    psychosocial nursing
    environment, 25
    health, 29
    nursing, 32
    person, 27

Language
    use and misuse of, 194
    see also Words
Laxative abuse, after childhood
    sexual abuse, 88–9
Learning
    experiential, 46–7, 165–6,
        210–21
    on the families unit, 211–13
    from practice, 193–4
    in seminars, 213–17
Leisure activities see Activities
Logic v. emotion, 43–7, 49–50
Lysis and scanning, 78

Main, Dr Tom, 18

Mastectomy, seminar case
    example, 157–8
Memory
    and abusive experiences, 119
    manageable doses, 122
    physical pain obliterating,
        121–4
    refusing to die, 128–30
    seminar case examples, 182–3,
        185–6
    suppressing, 120, 121
    of trauma, 125–6
    see also Body memories
Mental health nurses, desired
    skills, 63
Mental health nursing models,
    16–17, 63–4
Mental health placements,
    163–4
Mental illness
    NHS costs, 13–14
    prevalence, 13
    small units, 14
Metaparadigms, 23
Models see Nursing models

Nafsiyat (Intercultural
    Psychotherapy Centre), 208,
    209
National Health Service (NHS),
    reorganizations, 43
    policy documents, 60–1
'New nursing', 136, 138, 139
NHS see National Health Service
Nurse–patient relationship, 9–10,
    78–9
    biographical approach, 186
    boundaries, 136–8, 144
    involvement with patients,
        155–6

knowing the patient, 135, 136
ordinary activities and therapy,
    212
see also Privacy
Nurse–therapist relationship, 10
Nurses
    emotional work of, 45–6
    need for assertiveness, 193
    participation in management
        decisions, 49–50
    personal *v.* professional lives,
        192–3
    practice knowledge, 194
    presentational skills
        development, 193–4
    psychotherapeutic capacity,
        43–4
Nurses' Association for
    Psychodynamic
    Psychotherapy, 17
Nursing
    cultural influence on, 15
    v. medicine, status, 16
    profession *v.* craft, 18–19
    in psychosocial model of
        practice, 30–2
    see also Psychosocial nursing
Nursing case conferences, 193
Nursing models, 14–17
    assessment and comparison of,
        33
    autonomy paradigm, 34
    derived from practice, 19
    failure in practice, 15
    intervention model, 72–3
    makers *v.* users, 14–15
    in mental health, 16–17, 63–4
    private duty model, 54–5
    psychodynamic, 17–19
    types, 33

see also Cassel model;
    Psychosocial model of
    practice
Nursing process, rationality of?, 16

Objectivism, 44, 201
Observation, direct, 42, 44
    see also Ethnography
Older people
    ENB course, Nursing Elderly
        People, 178
    see also Biographical work with
        older people
Outcomes of psychosocial nursing
    see Goals and outcomes of
        psychosocial nursing

Pain
    body tissues as repositories of,
        121
    influenced by psychological
        factors, 126
    as language of body memories,
        120
    obliterating memories, 121–4
Parenting, 'good enough', 26, 96
Participant observation *see*
    Ethnography
Partnership
    *Patient Partnership: Building a
        Collaborative Strategy*, 64–5
    *Working in Partnership: a
        Collaborative Approach to
        Care*, 62–4
*Patient Partnership: Building a
    Collaborative Strategy*, 64–5
Patients
    as active participants, 7
    developing sense of
        responsibility, 10

Patients – *continued*
  own ways of extending therapy,
    132–3
  partnership with, 64–5
  see also Activities;
      Nurse–patient relationship;
      Privacy
Peplau, Hildegard, 17–18
Perfection, differing perspectives
    of, 206–7
Permissiveness, 10
Person, in psychosocial model of
    practice, 26–7
Phenomenology, 44–5
Philosophy of psychosocial nursing
  environment, 24
  health, 28
  nursing, 30
  person, 26
Physical activities, 76
Play, 78
Poetry reading, 76–7
Police and Criminal Evidence Act
    1984, 96
Policy guidelines
  child care, 96, 98
  NHS reforms, 60–1
Political correctness, 205
Positivism, 44
  see also Objectivism
Primary nursing, 57
Privacy
  appropriate, 143–5
  boundaries in nurse–patient
    relationship, 136–8, 144
  definitions, 139
  importance of, 140–2
  instrumental value of, 140–1
  and integrity, 142–3
  moral dimension to, 141–2

patient's right to, 139–40
  significance of, 139–45
Private duty nursing model, 54–5
Prohibition of Female
    Circumcision Act 1985, 96
Projection, 215–16
Psychoanalytical psychotherapy, 6,
    17–18
Psychodynamic Education Group,
    RCN, 17
Psychodynamic models of nursing,
    17–19
Psychosexual nursing, gaining
    recognition for, 160–2
Psychosexual Nursing Network,
    160
Psychosexual nursing seminars,
    152–62
  case examples brought to,
    154–5, 156, 157–8
  development of, 159–60
  with experienced nurses,
    153–5
  leader's role, 161, 219–21
  outcomes, 158–9
  regional programmes, 160
  student nurses, 161
  working with feelings, 157
Psychosocial care in the black
    community, 207–8
Psychosocial model of practice,
    22–32
  environment, 24–5
  health, 28–9
  interrelatedness of concepts,
    33–4, 34
  nursing, 30–2
  person, 26–7
  structure, 23
  see also Cassel model

Psychosocial nursing
  current practice, 9–10, 13–14
  development, 6, 8–9
  goals *see* Goals and outcomes of
    psychosocial nursing
  outcomes *see* Goals and
    outcomes of psychosocial
    nursing
  philosophy *see* Philosophy of
    psychosocial nursing
  practice, research and
    scholarship objectives, 35
  training, 8–9, 46–7
  see also Activities
Psychotherapy
  'black on black', 208
  intercultural, 208
  psychoanalytical, 6, 17–18

Racism *see* Black–white
    interactions; Blackness
Reality, concept of, 45
Re-enactment, 24
Reflection, 10, 165–6
Reflexivity, 45, 46–7
Remembering *see* Memory
Reminiscence
  satisfying or painful?, 180
  see also Biographical work with
    older people
Research
  action research, 19–21
  co-operative enquiry, 19–20
  direct observation, 42, 44
  enhancement approach, 20
  ethnography (participant
    observation), 44, 45, 46, 47–9,
    51
  reactions to researcher, 45
  see also Balint-style seminars,

research study; Cassel
    hospital research study
Resources, wastage of, 48–50

Self-destruction, 130–2
Self-esteem, encouraging, 77–8
Seminars
  examples, 214–19
  leader's role, 161, 219–21
  learning in, 213–17
  seminar training, 55
  see also Balint-style seminars;
    Psychosexual nursing
    seminars
Sexual abuse *see* Childhood sexual
    abuse
Shanti (Intercultural Women's
    Psychotherapy Service), 208,
    209
Shock, biological and emotional,
    125–8
Skills in psychosocial nursing *see*
    Knowledge, skills and
    attitudes
Social activities *see* Activities
Social enquiry, and subjective
    experience, 43–51
Social workers, in child protection
    work, 97, 100–1
  pitfalls for, 100, 101
  training, 97–8, 101
Soul murder, 120
Staff support
  child protection cases, 97
  childhood sexual abuse cases,
    89, 93
  and clinical supervision, 190–2
Stress, 31, 32, 130
Subjectivism, 44, 201
Supervision *see* Clinical supervision

232 Index

Support for nurses *see* Staff
    support

Therapeutic community principles,
    7–8
  programme, 10
Training *see* Education and
    training
Trauma, 120
  biological and emotional shock,
    125–8
  memory of, 125–6
  understanding defence
    mechanisms, 132–3
Treatment model, 71

Vision for the Future, 61–2
Voluntary space, 79–81

Words
  becoming lost, 120–1
  language use and misuse, 194
  power to wound, 121
  understanding through talk, 65
  use of, 59, 60
  as weapons, 120–1
Work/leisure, blurring of
    boundaries, 80–1
*Working in Partnership: a
    Collaborative Approach to
    Care*, 62–4